STRENGTH AND CONDITIONING FOR MIXED MARTIAL ARTS

TRAIN LIKE A PRO

Series Editor: Will Peveler

Rowman & Littlefield's Train Like a Pro series provides nonprofessional athletes, coaches, and trainers with training guides based on scientifically backed information that is both easy to follow and readily implemented. Each book covers the equipment, basic training physiology, specific training techniques, and tips for building a training plan for a specific sport, as well as competition, nutrition, and special considerations. These books are especially beneficial for athletes who have to train while working full-time jobs, as they provide recommendations for how training can be built around a busy schedule.

Strength and Conditioning for Mixed Martial Arts: A Practical Guide for the Busy Athlete by Will Peveler (2021)

Training for Mountain Biking: A Practical Guide for the Busy Athlete by Will Peveler (2021)

Training for Obstacle Course Racing: A Practical Guide for the Busy Athlete by Will Peveler (2021)

STRENGTH AND CONDITIONING FOR MIXED MARTIAL ARTS

A PRACTICAL GUIDE FOR THE BUSY ATHLETE

Will Peveler

ROWMAN & LITTLEFIELD
Lanham • Boulder • New York • London

Published by Rowman & Littlefield
An imprint of The Rowman & Littlefield Publishing Group, Inc.
4501 Forbes Boulevard, Suite 200, Lanham, Maryland 20706
www.rowman.com

6 Tinworth Street, London, SE11 5AL, United Kingdom

British Library Cataloguing in Publication Information Available

Library of Congress Cataloging-in-Publication Data

Names: Peveler, Will, author.
Title: Strength and conditioning for mixed martial arts : a practical guide for the busy athlete / Will Peveler.
Description: Lanham, Maryland : Rowman & Littlefield, 2021. | Series: Train like a pro | Includes index. | Summary: "A training guide for the nonprofessional mixed martial arts athlete, this book provides elite-level information that is easy to follow and readily implemented into a busy life schedule. It covers topics such as strength and conditioning, how to balance workouts with martial arts training, developing a training plan, nutrition, and more."—Provided by publisher.
Identifiers: LCCN 2020054118 (print) | LCCN 2020054119 (ebook) | ISBN 9781538139547 (cloth) | ISBN 9781538139554 (epub)
Subjects: LCSH: Mixed martial arts—Training. | Muscle strength. | Weight training.
Classification: LCC GV1102.7.M59 P49 2021 (print) | LCC GV1102.7.M59 (ebook) | DDC 796.81—dc23
LC record available at https://lccn.loc.gov/2020054118
LC ebook record available at https://lccn.loc.gov/2020054119

CONTENTS

ACKNOWLEDGMENTS

I would like to thank my wife, Renee, and our four sons, Grayson, Garrett, Will, and LJ, for supporting me throughout the process of writing this book, as well as the other books in the series. My wife was coerced into being in some of the photos, as well as taking some of the photos for the book. My son Grayson was also hijacked to take some of the photos as well. Without the support of my family I would not be able to do much of what I do.

I would also like to thank Justin Kilian for allowing me to yell into his office to ask questions and bounce training ideas off of him as I wrote this book. He provided an excellent sounding board for some of my programing ideas for *Strength and Conditioning for Mixed Martial Arts*.

I would like to thank Hayabusa Fightwear for providing photos for this book.

Last but not least, I would like to thank my editors, Christen Karniski and Erinn Slanina, for working with me during this process, putting up with all my questions, and making me sound somewhat intelligent.

INTRODUCTION

The goal of the Train Like a Pro series is to provide elite-level training information that is easily understandable and can be implemented in a very applicable manner. Each book in the series will provide you with information on the sport, required equipment and maintenance, a basic understanding of how the body responds and adapts to training, basic training principles, how to develop a training plan, exercise techniques, and basic sport nutrition for performance.

Most professional athletes are paid to both train and compete, and therefore their life is built around those work requirements. This series is written for the nonprofessional athlete. The majority of you reading these books have jobs, families, and other responsibilities that prevent you from working your life around training and competition. Instead you must find a way to work your training and competition into your life requirements. It is important to find a balance that allows you to work, have quality family time, and improve your performance.

The goal of *Strength and Conditioning for Mixed Martial Arts* is to provide you with the basic information that will allow you to be successful in the sport of mixed martial arts (MMA). This book was written with the beginner and novice in mind with a focus on equipment, training, nutrition, and competition. In short, it supplies the basic information I wish I would have had prior to starting my MMA training. This book focuses on MMA as a complete concept, combining various forms of martial arts to optimize combat performance. It is important to understand that fighting technique is not addressed in detail in this book. Instead the book focuses on strength and conditioning for improved performance. You cannot effectively learn fighting techniques through reading alone. It is important that you find a competent coach for that portion of your training. Whether you are training MMA for self-defense, as a hobby, for general fitness and health, or to fight in the cage, this book provides invaluable information that will improve your performance.

WHY BECOME INVOLVED IN MMA?

Enjoyment of the Sport

People become involved in MMA for various reasons. Most become involved for a combination of the reasons we will discuss. One of the primary reasons people become involved is that they love the sport and enjoy the mental and physical challenges that come with training. They look at MMA as a skill and art, and may have no desire to ever fight competitively.

Self-defense

Many people train MMA to better protect themselves in harmful situations. MMA provides individuals with the confidence to handle themselves in various circumstances. Regardless of an individual's rationale for participating in MMA, self-defense is a valuable tool.

Health and Fitness

Improved health is a great motivator for many who become involved in MMA during their pursuit of a healthier lifestyle. Individuals who are physically active are four times less likely to develop cardiovascular disease than those who do not participate in regular physical activity. This fact is so strongly supported by available research that the American College of Sports Medicine recently implemented the Exercise Is Medicine initiative, which is officially supported by the surgeon general.

MMA provides a challenging but attainable goal for those who wish to train for health or personal reasons. To maximize the health benefits of exercise, 30 minutes of physical activity per day is recommended for most days of the week. During training you will exceed those minimum recommendations and be well on your way to the development of a lifelong healthy lifestyle.

While physical activity has a strong positive impact on your health, you need to first ensure that you are healthy enough to begin an exercise program with no restrictions. Exercise takes your body out of homeostasis (the maintenance of balance within the human body: body temperature, blood glucose levels, etc.) and therefore increases the risk of a cardiovascular incident in those with undiagnosed or unknown heart conditions. You should seek a physician's clearance prior to beginning an exercise program to confirm that you are healthy enough to begin. This is especially true for sedentary individuals, older individuals, those who have not had a recent physical, and those who possess risk factors for the development of cardiovascular disease or signs of cardiovascular disease.

Competition

Some individuals become involved in MMA due to the competitive aspect. They enjoy pushing their body, mind, and resolve to the limits. Few sports will push you to the same limits as competing in MMA. Many fighters want to test their fighting skills against others to determine where they stand. The fighter with the best combination of skill, speed, power, strength, aerobic capacity, and anaerobic capacity is usually the fighter who wins.

HOW TO BECOME INVOLVED

It is important that you pick a great place to train, as it can either enhance your enjoyment of the sport or destroy it completely. Some training facilities are not beginner friendly and train too hard too often, ultimately turning people away. Other training facilities may be very good but may not focus on the fighting style that you are interested in. Look for a gym that is beginner friendly and well respected, and will easily align with your specific training goals. You will need to do a lot of homework prior to committing to a training facility. Most places allow free trials prior to making a commitment. Key concepts to consider when choosing a training facility are discussed in detail later in this book.

Many people train MMA to compete. If this is your goal, you should have a serious and focused discussion with your coach. This will allow your coach to develop your training plan so that you can optimally reach your goal. A good coach will not let you compete until they feel that you are ready.

Other than MMA, there are many different areas in which you may consider competing as you progress. One of the common areas that you may consider is jiujitsu. Competing in a jiujitsu tournament will allow you to focus on and develop your ground game. You can also choose to compete in boxing, kick-boxing, and Muay Thai to work on your stand-up. In each of these areas there are organizations that manage events and strictly regulate competitions.

GEAR FOR MIXED MARTIAL ARTS

Training for MMA requires specific gear to train and compete. This book provides information on the required equipment, how to choose the correct gear, and care and maintenance of that gear. Some of the gear discussed in this book includes gloves, hand wraps, mouthguards, shin guards, headgear, training pads, and fight wear/uniforms. While most gear will be similar across disciplines, some of the gear will be dependent on your precise style of training and the requirements of the facilities where you train.

TRAINING AND NUTRITION

To successfully participate in MMA, it is vital that you develop and maintain a sound training and nutrition plan. It is important to develop a plan that incorporates different volumes and intensities, along with appropriate recovery time, to optimize performance while preventing overtraining. As MMA requires aerobic capacity, anaerobic capacity, muscular endurance, muscular strength, muscular power, and flexibility, it is important to incorporate all these components into your training program. Most all individuals reading this book will have jobs, families, and other responsibilities, and these factors must be taken into consideration when developing a training program. This book will help you develop a basic training plan that will allow you to improve performance without overtraining.

While most mixed martial artists spend a lot of time developing their training plan, they commonly ignore their nutrition plan. To optimize training, you must not only eat specific types of food, but also consider the amount of food and the timing of meals. Your nutritional plan is just as important as our training plan.

1

TRAINING FACILITIES AND EQUIPMENT FOR MIXED MARTIAL ARTS

Training for mixed martial arts (MMA) requires the use of proper equipment and training facilities. This chapter provides advice on what to look for when choosing a gym for training. Every martial art has a specific name for their training facility (dojo, *dojang, wushu guan, kai muay*, studio, academy, etc.). To limit confusion, I use the terms *facility* and *gym* in this book. Every facility will have advantages and disadvantages; you must choose the facility that best suits your needs and goals.

This chapter also gives advice on how to choose the necessary equipment to start your MMA journey. Some of the equipment mentioned in this chapter will be necessary to start your training. Certain pieces of equipment will be nice but not required, while others will not be needed until you advance in your training. Learning what to look for when purchasing equipment will save you time and money, and possibly prevent injury. This chapter also discusses proper maintenance and care of your equipment.

TRAINING FACILITIES

One of the most important choices that you have to make is choosing the facilities in which you will train. The two main types of facilities that we will discuss are MMA gyms and strength and conditioning gyms. You may need to choose multiple gyms, depending on your goals and location. I currently train martial arts at The Edge Martial Arts, where they focus on Muay Thai, Gracie jiujitsu, and mixed martial arts. I conduct most of my strength and conditioning workouts in my home gym. You may choose to train stand-up at one facility, groundwork at another, and strength and conditioning at a third gym, or you may be lucky enough to train at a facility where you can conduct all your training in one place.

Cost is a factor that you must consider when choosing a training facility. Cost will vary greatly between facilities, and you will want to know the cost per month so that you can budget accordingly. While cost is a factor, keep in mind that you get what you pay for, and if you are serious about fighting you do not want to skimp on your training; however, there is not necessarily a strong correlation between cost and coaching level, and just because the cost is higher does not guarantee that the coaching is necessarily better. Most facilities require that you sign a contract. Make sure that you read the contract and know what you are committing to prior to signing.

Logistics is also a concern when choosing a training facility. If the drive or location is inconvenient, you may not train as often. This is one of the reasons that I have a home gym for my strength and conditioning sessions; however, I do drive 25 minutes one way for my MMA training, because the training I receive there makes it worth the drive. While not necessarily a deal breaker, it is a factor that you must consider.

Mixed Martial Arts Gym

Choosing an MMA gym can be daunting and intimidating for beginners. You will need to choose an MMA gym that best suits your needs and goals. Most gyms have free trials that will allow you to train to determine if it is a good fit. I suggest trying out a few gyms prior to committing to one. Also, most gyms allow a month-to-month contract if you need more time to decide. The month-to-month payment is typically higher per month than the contract price, but it allows you to try out the facility for a longer period of time before making a long-term commitment.

Another consideration when choosing a gym is the style of fighting. While many people argue about which style of fighting is the best, all styles have their strengths and weaknesses. MMA takes optimal techniques from all fighting styles to create an optimal fighter. MMA was built off the best of traditional martial arts. A large number of professional fighters started off in a traditional martial art and then transitioned into MMA. Many of you reading this book have probably followed the same path. But if you are interested in MMA as a combat sport, I would strongly suggest joining an MMA-specific gym, as the coaches there have already pulled the best techniques from various martial arts to create a complete program of study.

When choosing an MMA gym, you must also consider the overall philosophy, culture, and attitude of that gym. This is more important than you may believe. When you join a fight gym you are ultimately joining a family. You may not realize it in the beginning, but it is very true. Choose your family wisely. Stay away from gyms where the attitude and vibe are poor. Sit back and watch the interaction of everyone before, during, and after training. Moreover, there are gyms that have a spar hard philosophy and believe that you should spar hard every time you train. These gyms should be avoided. Hard sparring has a time and place but should be used sparingly. Choose a gym where hard sparring and egos are held in check by the participants and the coach.

One of the last things to consider is if the types of classes (Muay Thai, jiujitsu, sparring, etc.) the gym offers. Many facilities will have multiple different styles that they teach. You also must consider the availability of classes offered at that gym and if you will be able to fit them into your schedule. The gym can be an amazing gym yet not fit into your work and life schedule.

Workout Gyms

Few MMA gyms have a full workout facility for strength and conditioning; therefore, you may need to join a workout gym as well. When choosing a workout gym, there are few things you should consider. The first is that you will need to determine if they have the necessary workout equipment that you require for optimal training. There are some gyms that do not have free weights and others that may contain only free weights. Choose a gym with the mixture of free weights and machines that will allow you to accomplish your strength and conditioning goals. When choosing a gym, you also need to know what types of lifts are permitted. For example, some gyms do not allow dead lifts.

It is also important to know when the gym is open to determine if it will fit within your schedule. I advise visiting the gym during the primary time slot that you plan on training so you can determine if it is busy at that particular time. While you are visiting, make sure to ask when the high-traffic times are. High-traffic times typically extend your workout length, as there may be longer wait times on equipment.

If you are serious about strength and conditioning, and have the available space, you may want to consider building a home gym. This makes your strength and conditioning workouts more convenient. Considering that the average cost of a gym membership is about $600 per year (this is a conservative figure and will vary greatly by area), it may be a better idea to invest the money in a home gym. Building a home gym is not as expensive as you may believe. You can often find inexpensive secondhand equipment, as many people buy workout equipment, never use it, and then sell it at a significantly reduced rate. If you buy used equipment, always examine the equipment for any defects. As I have been physically active my entire life and plan on continuing for the remainder of my life, a home gym is a good investment for me. I also live in the country, and the closest gym is 25 minutes away. You will need to decide if a home gym is good investment for you.

If you decide to develop a home gym, you may also want to consider flooring. I divided my gym into a weight-training area and a fight training area. On the weight-training side, I use black horse stall mats for the floor, as they are durable and hard enough for the weights but provide some cushioning. Horse mats are also much less expensive per square foot in relation to gym flooring of the same durability. The downside of horse mats is that you will typically need to let them air out in your garage prior to putting them in the house due to the rubber smell that is common with the mats. Once they air out, the smell goes away.

On the fight side of my gym, I use a martial arts puzzle-type mat that is durable, provides cushioning, and is nonslip. If you choose to go this route, do not buy the inexpensive puzzle mats you find in common retail stores. These mats are not durable and will not last long. Purchase a mat that is specifically designed for martial arts. These mats will provide decent cushioning for falls and rolling but not takedowns. If you are going to be practicing takedowns or throws in your gym, you will need a grappling mat that provides much better protection.

FIGHTING GEAR

Gloves

A good pair of gloves is extremely important for training and is a piece of equipment you should not skimp on (see figure 1.1). Gloves serve two main purposes. First, they provide protection for your fingers, thumbs, hands, and wrists. Injuries to these areas are very common, and the risk can be decreased with a good pair of gloves and proper hand wraps. The second purpose of gloves is to provide protection for your sparring partners, which is why larger gloves are required when sparring. Naturally, competition gloves are designed primarily for protecting your fingers, thumb, hand, and wrist, and not your opponent. Whether you are buying a boxing glove, Muay Thai glove, MMA glove, or hybrid glove, there are certain aspects that you must consider.

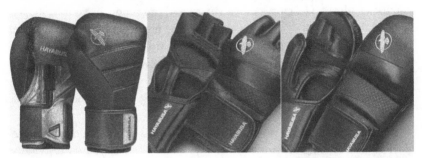

Figure 1.1. Muay Thai Gloves, MMA Gloves, and Hybrid Gloves. *Hayabusa Fightwear*

One of the first considerations is glove material. You can buy either leather or synthetic gloves. Leather versus synthetic is a highly debatable topic, and everyone has his or her own opinion. I am going to lay out the pros and cons for each, and you can decide for yourself which material works best for you. The first thing to keep in mind is that a poorly made glove is a poorly made glove, regardless of material. A well-made synthetic glove will outlast a poorly made leather glove. Leather is a long-lasting material when well maintained; however, it is important to note that while the leather itself may last a long time, the inner cushioning (foam, gel, etc.) will have a limited life span. Once the inner pads wear out, the glove is useless. Leather is also more breathable in relation to synthetic material and, therefore, is less prone to developing foul odors if properly maintained.

There are three basic types of synthetic gloves: vinyl, polyurethane (PU), and microfiber. Vinyl is tough and inexpensive, but vinyl is not very breathable, resulting in excessive sweating and a strong odor. PU gloves are not very resilient or breathable, resulting in early fatigue and strong odor. Microfiber is your best synthetic option. Microfiber gloves are sturdy, smooth, breathable, and odor resistant. Keep in mind that the quality of the glove will also determine how long the material holds up. I personally prefer leather, but microfiber gloves are my second choice.

Glove padding is another factor to consider when purchasing a pair of gloves. There are three basic materials used to pad gloves: foam, gel, and horsehair. In recent history, horsehair padding is typically only used in competition fighting gloves, as it transfers a lot of force into your opponent and offers little protection for your hands. Foam is the most common form of padding used in most modern gloves. Foam padding is lightweight and provides protection for both you and your sparring partner. Gel gloves are another option to consider when purchasing gloves. Gel gloves provide increased protection for your hands but increase the overall weight of the gloves. While not always the case, a typical 16-ounce gel glove can weigh in much higher than the advertised 16-ounce weight. The gel can create a glove that is front-heavy and hits hard. I have a set of gel gloves that I use for heavy bag workouts because of the added hand protection; however, I do not use them for sparring, as I feel they hit harder than my foam gloves.

Another consideration when purchasing gloves is fit and hand position. A glove should be snug but not tight. Always make sure that you try on a glove after your hands are wrapped so you can obtain a good feel of the fit. A glove should allow you to make a proper fist or as close as possible given the style of glove. Naturally, an MMA glove will allow a more proper fist in relation to a boxing glove.

One of the last considerations is closure and wrist support. There are two basic types of closures used in gloves. The first is lacing, and the second is Velcro. In the beginning, lace-up boxing gloves were your only option. With the invention of Velcro, everything changed; now professional boxers are about the only individuals who primarily use lace-up gloves. Lace-up gloves provide a more custom and tighter fit, allowing for excellent wrist support, but they require assistance to put on and take off, and prohibit quick glove removal. This would not be ideal for most training sessions, when you continuously switch from fighting to holding mitts/pads and then back with your partners. With modern Velcro gloves, the strap systems are designed to provide greater wrist support in relation to previous Velcro closures, and they are easy to get on and off. I advise staying with Velcro closure systems for most fighters and situations. Find a glove with a Velcro strap system that provides plenty of wrist support and is easy to get on and off.

Gloves will need to be replaced periodically. The typical life span of a glove is 8 to 12 months. This number is highly dependent on the volume and intensity of your training. There are various reasons that gloves need to be replaced periodically. One of the most important reasons is that the glove padding will break down throughout time, resulting in decreased protection for both your hands and your sparring partner. The two primary ways that most fighters notice that the padding has deteriorated is when their hands start to hurt more during bag rounds or their sparring partner points this fact out. Gloves should also be replaced when the material is torn or becomes rough, as it will cause abrasions to your sparring partner. Torn gloves can become less stable. The last primary reason to replace gloves is that when they develop a foul odor, it cannot be alleviated. You do not want to be the "stinky glove person" at your gym.

There are three basic types of gloves that you will need to consider purchasing for training and competition. There are other types of gloves, but these are the primary categories. Check with your instructor prior to purchasing gloves, as they may have requirements due to their specific training regimen and experience.

Boxing and Muay Thai Gloves

The first category that I will discuss is boxing and Muay Thai gloves. I put these gloves in the same category even though there are slight differences between the two types of gloves. In Muay Thai, you have to be able to work from the clinch; therefore, the glove is designed to allow you to open the hand slightly more than with a boxing glove. In addition, the thumb is typically not held as close to the hand as a boxing glove. Muay Thai gloves will typically have a pad down the side of the glove for blocking kicks and elbows. I have trained Muay Thai with both boxing and Muay Thai gloves, and found they both work well.

Overall considerations when purchasing gloves were mentioned earlier; however, there are other aspects to consider when purchasing boxing or Muay Thai gloves. One of those considerations is glove size and weight. As the glove weight increases, so too does the size and padding of the glove. Smaller gloves allow more force to transfer during a punch in relation to heavier gloves. Thus, smaller gloves are used during competition, as they produce more damage, and larger gloves are used in sparring and bag work, as they reduce damage to both the fighter's hand and his opponent. Smaller gloves also make it easier to slip punches past your opponent's defenses.

Gloves come in 8-, 10-, 12-, 14-, 16-, and 18-ounce sizes. The size that you need will be dependent on your size and the purpose of the glove. Boxing and Muay Thai competition gloves range from anywhere between 8- and 12-ounce gloves. Pro Muay Thai fights will use 8-ounce gloves for lighter weights and 10-ounce gloves for heavier weights. Amateur fights will typically use 10-ounce gloves for lighter fighters and 12-ounce gloves for heavier fighters. In most cases, 16-ounce gloves will be used for sparring. The use of heavier gloves provides more padding to protect your sparring partner. The exception is when working with smaller fighters, who may need to drop down to 14-ounce gloves, and large fighters, who may need to move up to 18-ounce gloves for sparring.

When working with kids, you may need to drop down to 8- to 10-ounce gloves due to the size of their hands. During heavy bag workouts, you should choose a heavier glove, 14 to 18 ounces, depending on your size, to protect your hands. Lighter gloves can be used while working the heavy bag when the focus is on speed and not power.

Ideally, you will want a pair of gloves for sparring and a pair of gloves for bag work. Heavy bag work will break down the glove padding much faster than sparring. You do not want to spar with a pair of gloves with broken-down padding, as it will transfer more force to your sparring partner.

MMA Gloves

Depending on your coach's training philosophy, you may not need MMA gloves to start training. You will find that most gyms will want you to have a pair of boxing or Muay Thai gloves and require that you wait on using MMA gloves until you are more advanced. Fighting MMA requires that you become comfortable using MMA gloves, and you will eventually work into using them. You will also find that even the pro fighters spend more time in boxing or Muay Thai gloves than they do in MMA gloves.

MMA gloves are designed for both striking and grappling. This requires that the gloves allow a wide range of motion for the hand, thumb, and all four fingers. The downside to this freedom of motion is that the thumb and fingers are more susceptible to damage, and accidental eye gouging can occur during training and competition. When purchasing gloves, make sure you have adequate movement.

MMA gloves typically come in small, medium, large, and extra large. You will need to determine the size of glove that best fits your hand. Make sure that you try on the gloves with your hands wrapped to see how they fit. MMA gloves typically come in 4- to 10-ounce weights. Competition MMA gloves are typically 4 to 6 ounces, and hybrid gloves typically range from 7 to 10 ounces.

Another type of glove you may want to consider is a hybrid glove. These gloves are designed similar to traditional MMA gloves but with greater padding. These gloves are used for easy sparring, as they provide greater padding than a traditional MMA glove but still allow for movement of the hand, thumb, and fingers for grappling. These gloves are lighter in weight and have less padding in relation to boxing or Muay Thai gloves; therefore, greater care must be taken during sparring.

Glove Maintenance

It is important to take care of your gloves to prolong their usable life span. One of the most important things to do is to make sure that your gloves are laid out to dry after each use. The biggest mistake beginners make is that they put their gloves in their gym bag after training and leave them there until they pull them out for the next session. This creates a wet environment that allows bacteria to grow.

Once you get home and pull your gloves from your bag, wipe them down inside and out with antibacterial wipes or vinegar and water. After cleaning, open up the gloves as much as possible so that air can circulate into them for better drying. I have a dehumidifier in my basement, and I set the gloves next to the dehumidifier after each use, and they dry quickly.

Another option is to use deodorizers designed for boxing gloves that slide into your gloves to wick away the moister and kill the smell. Glove deodorizers are typically bags filled with cedar chips that allow the moisture to easily pass into the bag and away from the glove.

The last option is to use a glove or boot dryer to allow air to flow into the glove to dry it. Glove dryers can be either electric, blowing air into and out of the glove, or nonelectric, holding the glove open and allowing air to easily flow into the glove.

Leather gloves should be wiped dry and then rubbed down with leather conditioner once they are clean and dry. This will prolong the life of the leather and keep it from becoming too dry and cracking.

Hand Wraps

When conducting pad work, bag work, or sparring, it is important to have your hands and wrists wrapped for protection. Heavy or repetitive punching can damage your hands and wrists. Wrapping the hands provides support to these areas and reduces the risk of injury. Wrapping hands protects the knuckles from abrasion, stabilizes the wrist, provides protection for the thumb, and wicks away sweat from the hands and gloves.

It is important to learn how to properly wrap the hands and wrists to provide optimal protection. When wrapping, it is important not to put the wrap on too tight. This will reduce circulation and may prevent you from making a proper fist. On page 10, I will talk you through a basic hand wrap. This is just one of many techniques used to wrap the hand, thumb, and wrist. You may need to find alternate ways that will work better for your specific hand.

When wrapping your hands, it is important that you do not wrap them too tightly or too loosely. It will take time and practice to get it correct. To accomplish this task, there are two basic principles you will want to follow. The first principle is that you want the wraps to be firm but not tight when wrapping. The second is that you want to keep the fingers spread and the muscles tight as you wrap so that when you relax, the wraps will be firm but not too tight. When you finish you should be able to make a comfortable fist with the hands and wrist firmly supported. Use the following steps:

- To wrap your hands, begin with the hand wrap rolled up so that the Velcro closure is on the inside of the wrap and the thumb loop is on the outside of the wrap with the writing "This Side Down" visible.
- Place your thumb through the loop and bring the wrap angled down the back side of the hand toward the wrist (opposite your thumb). The "This Side Down" label should be against your hand and not seen. At the wrist you will wrap around twice, ending at the thumb.
- Go upward across the back of the hand toward your 5th finger (fingers are numbered 1 to 5, starting with 1 at the thumb and ending with 5 at the little finger), and then wrap around the knuckles three times. On the third wrap you will end by the thumb. From this position you will go down and across the back side of the hand toward the wrist.
- Go around the wrist one and a half times, ending at the thumb.
- From the thumb, cross up the back of the hand and in between your 5th and 4th fingers, and onto the palm side of your hand.
- Wrap across the palm of your hand toward the thumb, around the knuckles, and back to the thumb.
- Once you reach the thumb, cross the back of your hand toward the wrist and complete one and a half wraps, ending at the thumb.
- From the thumb, cross up the back of the hand and in between your 4th and 3rd fingers, and onto the palm side of your hand.
- Wrap across the palm of your hand toward the thumb, around the knuckles, and back to the thumb.
- Once you reach the thumb, cross the back of your hand toward the wrist and complete one and a half wraps, ending at the thumb.
- From the thumb, cross up the back of the hand and in between your 3rd and 2nd fingers, and onto the palm side of your hand.
- Wrap across the palm of your hand toward the thumb, around the knuckles, and back to the thumb.

- Once you reach the thumb, cross the back of your hand toward the wrist and wrap around the wrist with the remaining wrap and close the Velcro fastener.
- On the palm side of your hand, take and wrap the edges of the wraps and wrap them underneath one another, forming a bar across the hand. This allows you to make a better fist in relation to leaving a wide wrap across your palm.

Hand Wrap Maintenance

Hand wraps should be warn only once and then cleaned prior to using them again. Hand wraps absorb a lot of sweat during training and are a breeding ground for bacteria. I keep enough sets of hand wraps so that I do not run out within a one-week training period. When washing hand wraps, it is important to fold the Velcro back on itself so that it does not attach to another hand wrap, creating a massive tangled mess during the washing cycle. Never throw a loose hand wrap into the washing machine, as it will wrap around everything, including the washing machine's agitator. Instead, place the hand wraps in a mesh laundry bag that can be zipped closed to prevent the wraps from coming out and wrapping around the agitator.

Mouthguards

Another important piece of equipment that you will need is a mouthguard. While everyone knows that a mouthguard is designed to protect your teeth, many do not know that it does a lot more than just protect teeth from damage. The mouthguard also provides a degree of protection for the soft tissues of your mouth and tongue. A good mouthguard will also dissipate impact by acting as a shock absorber, reducing stress on the jaw. It is often stated that mouthguards reduce the occurrences of concussions; however, to date, there is no strong scientific evidence that concussive forces to the brain are lessened due to the use of mouthguards.

There are two basic categories of mouthguards that you can purchase. The first choice is boil-and-bite mouthguards. These mouthguards are relatively inexpensive and easy to mold. There is a large variety of options for boil-and-bite mouthguards, and you may need to do a little research to determine which is best for you. Make sure that you purchase a mouthguard designed specifically for MMA, as mouthguards designed for another sport will not protect optimally.

Custom mouthguards are your next option. This option is more expensive but provides greater protection. Between boil-and-bite and custom, I prefer custom mouthguards for both fit and protection. Custom mouthguards can be purchased through your dentist or directly from a lab. When purchasing directly from a lab, they will send you the necessary supplies and directions to make a mold of your teeth. Once the mold is made, you ship it back to the company, and they make your mouthguard. This option is substantially less expensive in relation to going to the dentist, but a dentist will be able to take the mold and ensure the mouthguard fits properly. I have used both dentist and lab mouthguards, and both worked just as well. As I have no dental issues or concerns, I will continue to purchase directly from a lab.

Regardless of which you choose, make sure the mouthguard fits properly. The mouthguard should fit snuggly to your top teeth without falling out when you open your mouth. You should be able to talk and breathe relatively comfortably, given that you have a mouthguard in. If your mouthguard is not comfortable, you will not wear it regularly. Those with braces will need a double-sided mouthguard designed specifically for braces. Lastly, it is always advisable to talk to your dentist about a mouthguard for MMA, regardless of which route you choose.

Mouthguard Maintenance

It is important to clean your mouthguard after each use. Leaving your mouthguard in your bag without cleaning it is a guaranteed method of growing your own bacteria. You can clean your mouthguard by brushing it with toothpaste, letting it soak in mouthwash, or cleaning it with denture cleaner (denture cleaner may be too harsh for some mouthguards).

Headgear

Headgear is designed to decrease the impact of strikes, reducing the rate of head injury. Headgear may be required when sparring or competing depending on the philosophy of the gym where you train and the rules of the competitions you choose to enter. If you are required to wear headgear during a competition, it is a good idea to train in similar headgear so you can become accustomed to the altered field of vision; however, headgear is no longer a requirement in many combat sport competitions and never required in MMA competitions.

The use of headgear is highly debated at every level of combat sports. On the surface, it seems as though added head protection is a good idea and that everyone should wear headgear when sparring, especially given the high rate of concussions in combat sports. But in most cases, it is the acceleration of the head following a punch that results in brain trauma, and headgear may not protect against that particular type of acceleration. It is the acceleration of the brain within the skull during impact that results in concussion. When looking at the forces exerted on the brain from a strike, those forces can be either linear (along a line) or angular (rotational). The angular force that occurs during rotation (a hook) is much more likely to result in a concussion in relation to linear forces (a jab).

It is also theorized that wearing headgear during sparring results in the fighter taking more risk and the opponent throwing punches faster and harder because of the perceived added protection of the headgear. When you put on headgear to spar, many individuals believe you are well protected and therefore can take much harder hits. Wearing headgear also limits the fighter's view, resulting in more punches and kicks landed. Wearing headgear makes your head a much larger target.

While protection from concussion is highly debated, there are distinct advantages to wearing headgear while sparring. Headgear has been shown to decrease the risk of facial lacerations, and there is a decreased risk of a broken nose when wearing headgear with a bar or a full-cage helmet.

My goal is not to dissuade you from using headgear, but instead to educate you on the mechanics of concussions and that headgear does not offer the level of protection that many believe it does. It is important that you and your sparring partner understand that the headgear is there as backup for the misjudged strikes and not an open invitation to hit faster and harder. I believe headgear is a good idea for harder sparring sessions, keeping in mind that it does not add the level of protection that many believe it does.

There are a few things to consider when purchasing headgear. If headgear is required at your gym, ask the instructor what is required prior to purchasing headgear. They may have specific requirements for their gym. Headgear comes in the same materials as gloves, and you should choose the most optimal material that fits your budget. Headgear should fit snug and should not move around on your head, but it also should not be so tight that it is uncomfortable to wear. There is nothing worse than catching a cross and then seeing nothing but the inside of your helmet because it twisted on your head and you are trying to look out the ear hole.

There are three primary styles of headgear to choose from: open face, closed face, and full cage. Open-face headgear allows for the greatest field of view but provides little to no face protection. Closed-face headgear provides greater protection for the face and covers the range of headgear, with cheek protection to headgear with a face bar. The downside to closed-face gear is that it limits your field of vision. Full-cage headgear has a padded helmet with a full cage protecting the face. This type of headgear is more commonly found in traditional-style marital arts.

Headgear Maintenance

Maintenance of sparring headgear is similar to the process you would use for gloves. When sparring is completed, make sure to wipe down your headgear with antibacterial wipes and dry it thoroughly. If your headgear is leather, you will need to wipe it down periodically with leather conditioner.

Shin Guards

Shin guards are used to protect the soft tissue of the anterior portion of your leg and dorsal surface of the foot. Think of them as boxing gloves for your legs. When throwing certain kicks, the tibia (shin bone) is often used as the striking surface. When the shin makes contact with a hard surface, for example, your opponent's shin, it can be very painful. Shin guards provide protection by decreasing the impact of those strikes. I always spar with shin guards, as it allows me to more comfortably check kicks and throw lower body or leg kicks that could be checked by my opponent. When sparring, it is quite common to catch your opponent's elbow when they bring their arm in close to their body to block your body kick. Catching an elbow on the shin or top of the foot can be painful even through the pads and can result in a fracture to the bones of the feet. Wearing shin guards will also make your strikes more comfortable (I use this term loosely) for your sparring partner. I also recommend shin guards for beginners for bag work until their shins become more conditioned. This allows them to focus on technique, instead of pain, when throwing hard, fast kicks.

Shin guards are available in the same materials (leather and synthetic) as gloves and should be given the same consideration when making a purchase. When choosing shin guards, you will need to find the combination of protection and mobility that works best for you. As the padding increases, mobility will slightly decrease. Shin guards for MMA will have more mobility but provide slightly less foot protection, whereas shin guards made for stand-up fighting have more padding but less mobility. Shin guards will typically come in small, medium, and large. As sizes will vary between manufacturers, make sure to consult the sizing chart prior to making a purchase to ensure a good fit.

Shin Guard Maintenance

Maintenance for shin guards will also be similar to the process you would use for gloves. When sparring is completed, make sure to wipe down your shin guards with antibacterial wipes and thoroughly dry them off. If your shin guards are made of leather, you will need to wipe them down periodically with leather conditioner.

Groin Protectors

During sparring sessions, it is not uncommon to receive kicks to the groin area, especially when leg kicks are allowed. This makes groin protection vitally important. For males, groin protection is also required for all stand-up and MMA fights. Groin protection requirements for females vary depending on the stand-up genre and the particular commissioning body of the tournament. For stand-up fights, female requirements range from required to prohibited. During jiujitsu tournaments, groin protection is prohibited for both genders, as the hard surface gives advantage for certain techniques, for instance, arm bars.

When choosing groin protection there are a few things to consider. First and foremost is the amount of protection provided by the groin protector. Second is comfort and mobility. It can be difficult to find a groin protector that adds optimal protection but is comfortable to wear. Certain body types may benefit by mixing brands (protector from one brand and holder from another) to achieve optimal protection, comfort, and mobility. For females, it is even more difficult due to the limited options currently available.

Groin Protection Maintenance

Make sure to wash the protective cup holder after each use, just as you would any other piece of clothing. You can hand wash the protective cup with water and soap, and let it dry for the next use.

Women's Chest Protectors

Female chest protectors are used to shield the female breast when competing or sparring in striking events. The choice to use chest protectors during sparring is highly personal, as some female breasts can be more sensitive than others. Chest protection is often required during competition. If chest protectors are required for a fight in which you are competing, it is a good idea to spar a few rounds wearing yours during training to make sure there are no unforeseen issues with fit and comfort.

Most female chest protectors are designed similar to sports bras but have a pocket that allows you to slide in a protective cup. The protective cups are made of materials that vary from hard plastic to dense foam. Both the sports bra and cups come in varying sizes. It is important to find a combination that is comfortable, as well as protective.

Women's Chest Protector Maintenance

Make sure to wash the sports bra after each session using the manufacturer's recommendation. If you have removable protective cups, make sure to remove them prior to putting the sports bra into the washing machine. Most protective cups can be hand-washed with water and soap.

Fight Wear

When fighting and training there will be specific clothing that may be required. Always ask your coach prior to buying any gear. For example, only white gi are permitted where I train. Had I not asked, it would have been an issue, as I am not a fan of white and would have purchased any color other than white. Each competition will have specific regulations on required attire, and you will need to make sure you meet those requirements. In the following sections I will discuss some of the basics of fight wear.

Fight Tops

For male fighters, tops are not permitted in most fighting events and therefore are not an issue; however, it is common, and often required, to wear shirts during training sessions for stand-up training and sparring. Choose a shirt material that is made from synthetic fibers (primarily polyester) that are specifically woven in a manner that allows moisture transfer from the skin and evaporation of sweat to occur. This will keep you cooler during training sessions. The difference between a poorly made synthetic fiber shirt and a well-made synthetic fiber shirt is the shape of the individual fibers and alignment of the fiber. Nonetheless, keep in mind that synthetic fibers more readily grow bacteria and thus will smell after a period of time even with thorough washing.

Because of this, some individuals choose to train in cotton or cotton blend shirts. When training in a climate-controlled environment, heat dissipation may not be a large concern.

Female fighters will typically train in a shirt worn over a sports bra or a sports bra alone. Females should consider wearing a sports bra to provide support and limit chafing during training. Due to the nature of MMA, the breast will move a lot, and the larger the breast the greater the need for support. A sports bra differs from a normal bra, in that it will typically fit comfortably snug, is made of synthetic material for wicking, and possesses a band along the bottom to help hold it in place. Do not get hung up on looks and concentrate more on support and comfort. Keep in mind that this advice is coming from a guy giving coaching advice and not a female who has firsthand experience with the topic.

Fight Shorts

You will need shorts designed specifically for MMA, as there are distinct differences between MMA shorts and other shorts. If you are only doing stand-up with no groundwork, then Muay Thai shorts, boxing shorts, or kickboxing shorts are fine; however, if you are doing no gi groundwork or stand-up, it makes more sense to buy a pair of MMA shorts for both.

MMA shorts are designed for both stand-up and groundwork. Never wear shorts with pockets, as toes or fingers can easily be caught in the pocket during grappling. There should also never be any metal parts (buttons, zippers, metal eyelets, etc.) on the shorts, as they can cause abrasions or lacerations. A good pair of MMA shorts will have elastic material in the groin area to allow a full range of motion without binding. There will also be slits located to the outside of each leg so as not to impede movement when kicking. The waist will have a drawstring and Velcro closures to ensure that the shorts do not slip down during grappling.

A pair of compression shorts for MMA is another consideration. Compression shorts allow for smoother movement when grappling; stay in place better, which will decrease mat rash; and have the added advantage of compression. The downside to compression shorts is that they hide nothing, and guys should remember this if they are not wearing groin protection. Oftentimes fighters will wear compression shorts under their MMA shorts to gain the benefits of both. Compression shorts are also recommended for wearing under your gi to prevent friction rash and hold everything in place when not wearing groin protection.

Gi

A gi is a martial arts uniform that is often used when training jiujitsu. The gi uniform consists of a top that folds over itself in the front to close, a belt to signify rank and hold the top closed, and a pair of pants with a drawstring. Jiujitsu gi are much thicker in relation to gi worn in other traditional martial arts to hold up to the stress of grappling.

When choosing a jiujitsu gi, it is important that you choose a gi that is sturdy enough to hold up during training and competition. Thickness of the gi is one thing you must consider. Thicker gi make it harder for your opponent to get a good grip and therefore gives you an advantage during competition; however, they are much hotter than lightweight gi. Individuals who compete in jiujitsu often have lightweight gi for training and heavyweight gi for competition. Speak to your coach about what is required at your gym prior to purchase.

Gi Maintenance   Keeping a gi clean, especially a white one, is a challenge in and of itself. It is recommended to avoid using bleach, as it will damage the gi. Instead, it is recommended to spot clean stains and then wash in a mixture of vinegar and baking soda in cold water. When washing, set your machine for about a 30-minute soak. Always wash your gi in cold water, as hot water will cause significant shrinkage.

Do not machine dry your gi, as it will cause the gi to shrink each time you dry it. There is more than one guy where I train who walks around in gi bottoms that end at least five inches above the ankle. But if your gi is slightly too large you can dry it in order to shrink it to fit. If you do choose to shrink your gi in the drier, pull it out periodically to see how much it has changed in size, as opposed to leaving it in until completely dry and having it shrink too much.

Rash Guards

Rash guards are designed to help prevent mat burn, gi burn, and the transfer of bacteria. When working no-gi jiujitsu, it is important to wear a rash guard to prevent your skin from sliding across the mat, creating a burn as a result of the friction between your skin and the mat. Rash guards also help with reducing sweat transfer while rolling. Although not permitted in every competition, wearing a rash guard under your gi is beneficial, as it provides an extra layer of protection.

Rash guards take a lot of punishment, and you will need to buy a rash guard that will hold up during training. Rash guards are built differently in relation to compression shirts, and most compression shirts will not hold up to the rigors of rolling. You will also want to find a rash guard that is somewhat breathable so heat can easily dissipate from your body. A nonbreathable rash guard under your heavy gi top makes for a very hot and miserable training session.

Pads

While there are various pads that you will use for training in MMA, I am just going to focus on the two primary sets you will need: focus mitts and Thai pads. Learning how to properly hold focus mitts and Thai pads is a skill in and of itself, and it takes a lot of practice. It is important that you learn how to hold correctly to optimize performance and minimize the risk of injury.

Many gyms will have communal focus mitts and Thai pads that you can use when training. Some gyms, however, require that you purchase your own. I prefer to have my own pair, as opposed to using a communal pair that everyone uses. I am not a germophobe, but it is very difficult to keep communal focus mitts as clean as I would like. Moreover, the pads supplied by the gym are, or will be, worn out, and you will feel every kick and punch through the pads.

When purchasing pads, you want to purchase pads that give you a good combination of padding and mobility. Pads come in the same materials discussed earlier with boxing gloves, and those same factors should be taken into consideration when purchasing pads. You want to purchase pads that feature good padding to provide protection from hard punches and kicks. Make sure to read reviews prior to purchasing.

Focus Mitts

Focus mitts fit on your hands and are designed to catch punches when working with a partner. They allow you and your partner to flow smoothly while working on striking drills that more closely resemble competition. The pad holder will be moving in a fighting stance using correct footwork and occasionally throw punches with the pads for response drills.

Thai Pads

Thai pads are elongated pads that run the length of your forearm, providing protection as you catch kicks and punches. The benefit of using Thai pads is that you can flow similar to sparring. The pad holder can work on his footwork and throw occasional punches and kicks to initiate response drills.

Pad Maintenance

Cleaning and care of striking pads is similar to glove maintenance. Be aware that pads will wear out throughout time, resulting in decreased protection, and need to be replaced periodically. Do not use torn or damaged pads, as they could fail during training.

Bags

Training bags allow you to work on the power, speed, and accuracy of your strikes. There are numerous different bags that serve different purposes. In this discussion I only focus on the basic categories of bags you will most likely be using in your training. Within each category there are numerous variations. It is beneficial to have a bag or two at your house to train when not at your gym.

Heavy Bags

Heavy bags are large punching bags that typically weigh between 50 and 150 pounds; however, you can get heavier or lighter bags. There are a few factors to consider when choosing the correct weight. The first factor is your own weight. As your opponent will most likely be close to your weight, it makes sense to purchase a bag that is as close to your weight as possible. The second consideration is where you intend to hang the heavy bag. You need to make sure it can support the weight of the bag without causing damage to the structure you are hanging the bag from. The last consideration is the heavier the bag, the harder it will be on your hands and legs. If you are willing to do some work, you can purchase an unfilled heavy bag and stuff it to meet both your weight and hardness requirements.

There are many different types of heavy bags, and you will need to choose the style that works best for your current level of training. A good all-around bag for MMA is a Muay Thai bag. Muay Thai bags are typically six feet tall, allowing for low, mid, and high kicks when training. Muay Thai bags are also smaller in circumference in relation to traditional bags. This allows you to kick the bag with your shins and avoid your foot catching on the back side of the bag, as it would with a larger circumference bag.

Traditional heavy bags are shorter and typically range anywhere between 42 and 52 inches in length, which eliminates low kicks. Traditional bags are typically much larger in circumference in relation to Muay Thai bags. While this does vary greatly among bags, Muay Thai bags do tend to be much harder than most heavy bags. In my home gym I have a 150-pound Muay Thai bag that I use when I am focusing primarily on kicks and a 150-pound traditional bag that is much softer, which I use when focusing on hands. I also have a freestanding bag, with a water base, that I use when I want to focus on technique and speed, as it is much easier on my hands.

A heavy bag is a piece of equipment for which I prefer synthetic material rather than leather, as breathability is not a concern. Vinyl and other synthetics provide alternatives that are tough and require less care in relation to leather. They are also less expensive in relation to leather heavy bags.

When hanging a heavy bag, always make sure the structure can handle the weight of the bag, keeping in mind that the bag will accelerate and jump when kicked or punched. An improperly hung bag can damage property and cause injury. If possible, avoid heavy-bag stands, as the legs of the stand will impede movement when working the bag. It is ideal to place the heavy bag so that you can work full circle around the bag, but this may not be feasible given your work space.

Speed Bags

A speed bag is a piece of equipment that is often misunderstood by beginners. Speed bags are designed to work on hand–eye coordination, speed, timing, and upper body muscular endurance. They are not designed to throw normal punches or develop power. Learning to properly use a speed bag takes time and practice. It is all about setting up your rhythm.

When choosing a speed bag, make sure to purchase one that has a sturdy base so that the bag responds in a predictable manner. A base that moves around a lot will make it extremely difficult to establish a rhythm. A good swivel is needed so that the bag moves freely and predictably. Changing the swivel on your speed bag will go a long way toward improving the performance of the bag. If more than one individual will be using the speed bag, you will need to purchase one that allows the height to be easily adjusted so the bag height is correct for the individual using it.

Double-End Bags

A double-end bag is a small bag that attaches to the ceiling and floor. The double-end bag is designed to work on your hand–eye coordination, speed, and accuracy. It requires you to make contact with a moving target. When punching a double-end bag, you must make smaller movements, as opposed to a heavy bag, where you are often working on power punches and calculated ranged attacks. The double-end bag will also give you an idea of what it feels like when you miss a punch.

A double-end bag is constructed similar to a speed bag but will have cords on both ends of the bag so it can be attached to the floor and ceiling. When installing a double-end bag on the floor, I recommend using an anchor bag that is specifically designed for that purpose. If you accidentally hit your toe on the anchor bag, it will be more forgiving in relation to something that is much more solid.

Shoes

While gyms prohibit wearing shoes on the mat, there are various situations where specialized shoes are required. The two primary types of shoes you will need to consider are running shoes and weight-training shoes. Each shoe is specifically designed to increase performance and decrease the risk of injury. During training, you will be working aerobic capacity, anaerobic capacity, and resistance. If you are training boxing or wrestling as part of your MMA program, you will need to look into shoes for each of those sports as well. In the following paragraphs I explain what to look for when purchasing running shoes and weight-training shoes.

Running Shoes

A good pair of shoes can make all the difference in the world. Running in improper shoes can not only be uncomfortable, but also result in the development of overuse injuries. One of the common questions I receive from beginning runners deals with leg pain, primarily in the region of the lower leg (ankle, shin, and knee). After a short consultation there are two common factors that are typically uncovered. The first concerns the individual increasing intensity or duration too quickly, which is easily modified through altering their training schedule (which usually means developing one). The second concern typically deals with the fact that they are running in improper shoes. Some common issues with shoes are as follows:

- Running in shoes that are not designed for running, for example, court shoes. Court shoes, for instance, basketball shoes, are designed to for making quick lateral movements on a court surface, whereas running shoes are primarily designed for forward movement only. Due to this fact, court shoes make a poor choice for running shoes.

- Training in running shoes that are old and well past their usefulness. The old running shoes that you have been mowing the yard in for the last three years are not a good choice for training.
- Running in new shoes that are not designed for your particular biomechanics. Running in new shoes that are not made for your intended purpose can lead to overuse injuries.
- Running in shoes that do not fit correctly. Running in shoes that do not fit properly can result in injury.

When purchasing running shoes, it is important to choose shoes that best fit your needs, budget, and, most importantly, individual anthropometrics and biomechanics. There are two key factors when choosing the type of shoe you wish to run in. The first deals with the manner in which you run, and the second concerns your weight. As an individual's weight increases, the need for cushioning will increase as well.

The interaction of the foot and the ground is extremely important with regard to running. While there are many variations, there are three basic categories that runners fall into: in-line (foot following the normal path from heel to toe while running), overpronation (foot excessively rolling toward the midline of your body), or supination (foot excessively rolling away from the midline of your body).

In-line or neutral runners follow the basic outline of the stance phase (when the foot is in contact with the ground) with little variation. They typically have a normal arch and do not excessively pronate. Due to this, a neutral-cushion shoe is recommended for these runners. A neutral-cushion shoe will provide cushioning and be built on a semicurved sole.

Overpronators deviate from the norm through excessive pronation during the mid-stance phase. Normal pronation that occurs during the mid-stance phase is the body's natural mechanism for absorbing the ground reaction forces to prevent injury. But when the foot overpronates, it alters running kinematics and can lead to overuse injuries in runners. A motion-control shoe that provides medial support and is built on a straight sole is designed to best address overpronation. Those that slightly overpronate may be better served in a stability shoe that provides slight medial support. While this recommendation appears straightforward, the reality is much more complicated. The typical cause of overpronation is lack of a normal arch; however, lack of flexibility and muscular imbalances or muscle weakness can also lead to overpronation. It is important to understand the cause of the overpronation to best address the problem. While a motion-control shoe will assist those who overpronate due to lack of a normal arch, it may not help if the overpronation is caused due to lack of flexibility, muscular weakness, or muscular imbalances.

Individuals who supinate (run on the outside of the foot) will typically have a high arch, which forces the foot to the outside as they run. A cushioned shoe built on a curved sole is ideal for supinators. The curved sole and lack of medial support encourage the foot to pronate during the stance phase.

There are key points to look for in a proper fit. The first is that you should have a thumb's width between your big toe and the end of the shoe. This measurement will need to be conducted while standing. With the shoes tied, the shoe should fit comfortably snug across the top of your foot (not tight). The last thing to check is to walk around to determine if the back of the shoe slips up and down significantly on the heel of your foot. If the heel excessively slides up and down, the shoe is too large. Also keep in mind that shoes from different brands may fit differently. If one brand does not fit correctly on your foot, try another. I have even experienced two different models of shoes from the same company fitting differently. One model fit the same as most shoes I run in, and a second model was narrow and tight in the toe box. Prior to running in your new shoes, I recommend wearing the shoes around the house for a few hours to determine if they are truly comfortable. This way you can return the shoes for another size or brand. Some running stores will have treadmills set up in the store and allow you to walk or run in the store prior to purchasing the shoes.

It is an unfortunate fact that running shoes wear down and must be replaced somewhat frequently. Not only does the sole wear thin and lose traction, but also the EVA material (the white cushioning material) becomes compressed and loses the ability to absorb ground reaction forces. The typical recommendations are to replace running shoes every 300 to 500 miles. The actual miles will vary due to the quality of the shoe, mass of the individual, intensity of the miles put on the shoes, and conditions the individual runs in; however, as long as the shoe is safe and comfortable there is no reason to purchase new shoes.

Shoes for Weight Training

There are a few variables to consider when determining shoes for your resistance training. You want to avoid lifting in your running shoes for two primary reasons. The first is that running shoes have cushioning that will depress significantly during a heavy lift, resulting in loss of stability. The second is that you do not want to prematurely wear down your running shoes. It is not the end of the world if you lift in your running shoes, but it is less stable and will decrease the life of your running shoes.

You also do not necessarily want a true weight-training shoe. Weight-training shoes have a thinner and much firmer sole with harder material (plastic or wood) at the heel of the shoe. This creates a much more stable platform when conducting movements that require pushing against the ground. It also allows you to better attain proper form for certain lifts. But powerlifting is not the goal of your training, and these shoes would be overkill. They are also too stiff to comfortably perform plyometrics or sprints.

A cross-training shoe is an ideal shoe for the type of weight training you will be conducting. A cross-training shoe will provide a strong base of support if you are doing heavy lifts, for example, squats or dead lifts, and enough mobility to comfortably conduct plyometrics or sprints. Shoes designed for cross-training will be built similar to a true weight-training shoe but with a few small differences. The cross-training shoe will have a little more cushion than a weight-training shoe but not as much as a running shoe. The heel will be firm but not as firm as a weight-training shoe, providing more flexibility.

Heart Rate Monitors

It is vitally important to monitor and control workout intensity during endurance training, and heart rate is an excellent tool for monitoring intensity. While you can measure pulse rate with your fingers and a watch, it is not as accurate and convenient as using a heart rate monitor to measure heart rate. For those who are serious about training, I recommend purchasing a heart rate monitor.

A heart rate monitor consists of a transmitter and a receiver. The transmitter fits around the thoracic region just below the pectoralis major. When placing the transmitter below the chest it is important to center the transmitter midline. The transmitter should be tight enough to remain still but not so tight as to be uncomfortable. The transmitter should be wet and placed against the skin to pick up the electrical impulse of the heart contractions. The receiver acquires the signal from the transmitter and displays heart rate. The receiver is typically worn on the wrist as a watch. With modern technology there are specific apps that allow you to link your smartphone with the transmitter and use your phone as the receiver.

The heart rate monitor will possess various functions that are useful for maintaining intensity and evaluating performance. Heart rate monitors vary in price based on function ($40 to more than $300). An entry-level heart rate monitor that provides heart rate and time will start at about $40. I recommend purchasing a heart rate monitor that at least has zone alarms. This will allow you to set alarms that sound when you go below (typically not a problem) or above (usually the problem) your training zone for the day. If you are going to train in a group, you need a heart rate monitor that is coded so that you do not pick up another athlete's heart rate as you train.

Instead of buying a complete system, you can by a heart rate strap with Bluetooth capabilities so that it can be paired with your smartphone. There are very good applications that are free or at minimum cost that you can download onto your phone. These applications will provide GPS data, as well as heart rate data. For many people, this will be the most affordable and viable option, as you most likely already own a phone. This allows you to track not only heart rate, but also distance traveled, speed, and grade. Once your workout is complete, you can then analyze the data. As a coach, I find this feature invaluable. I can examine my athlete's heart rate in relation to alterations in grade, speed, and distance during endurance training. One downside to using your phone for training in the cold is that the cold can quickly drain your battery during the winter months. I have had my phone shut down during a run even though I started the run with 100 percent battery life.

Another option is to purchase an entry-level GPS/heart rate monitor system. These units are a valuable training tool and start at about $100. Once you complete your workout, you can download the data to a computer or smartphone for evaluation. I own a GPS/heart rate monitor system but no longer use it, as I find my phone and apps to be more convenient and just as accurate.

When choosing a heart rate monitoring tool there are other options that you can consider, but these are the basics. One last thing to mention is that I have seen many athletes spend a lot of money on heart rate monitors but then never really use them. At that point, the heart rate monitor just becomes an expensive toy as opposed to a powerful training tool. Before purchasing an expensive heart rate monitor, really think about how you will integrate the system into your training program.

Punch Trackers

Punch trackers are accelerometers that connect to your smartphone and allow you to track your punches. The accelerometers are placed in your hand wraps at the wrist, where they can easily track movement, calculate velocities, and measure distances traveled. From the gathered data you will be able to determine the number of punches thrown; power and velocity of each punch; and, to a small degree, the type of punch thrown. They are great tools for determining training volume during sparring or a bag workout. The downside to the punch-tracking system is that they are currently unable to track kicks, knees, or elbows.

Where to Purchase Equipment

Unfortunately, there are few local stores that specialize in fighting gear; therefore, it is unlikely that you will have a local shop within driving distance. On occasion, local MMA gyms will provide equipment for sale, but they usually have limited inventory. If you are lucky enough to have a local fight shop, I strongly recommend that you pay it a visit. One of the benefits of buying from a local store is that you can try on equipment for fit and comfort prior to buying. A local store will also have experts who can help you make educated decisions. While everyone can gain invaluable equipment information from visiting a local fight store, it is even more important for those who are new to the sport.

Most of you will purchase equipment online. When shopping online there are a few things to consider. First and foremost is the return policy. Prior to purchasing equipment, educate yourself on the shop's return policies. Most online shops will allow you to try on equipment and return the item if it does not fit or simply does not work for you; however, very few online shops allow you to return equipment if you used the piece of gear during training. Understanding what is returnable and not returnable, and the conditions for returning an item, will save you money in the long run.

Another consideration is the knowledge level of the online sales staff. Most places hire workers who have a background in fighting so they can better answer your questions. If the person you are speaking with cannot answer your questions, politely ask to speak to someone else.

Whether you purchase your gear locally or online, always look up reviews on the gear you plan on purchasing. I advise looking at not only video and written reviews of the product, but also consumer reviews. When examined as a whole, consumer reviews typically provide relatively nonbiased feedback based solely on personal experience. Moreover, speak with your coaches and other members of the gym to see what they like and what experiences they have had with specific gear, local shops, and online shops.

2

BASIC TRAINING PRINCIPLES, PHYSIOLOGY, AND PSYCHOLOGY

This chapter provides the necessary training background required to better determine how you will plan and implement your training program for mixed martial arts (MMA) training. To create and adhere to a quality training program it is important that you understand how your body will respond to the stress applied during training and competition. The body responds to stress in very predictable ways, which allowed for the development of the training principles discussed in this chapter. Gaining an understanding of these basic principles will allow you to develop a sound training program and make better training choices.

BASIC TRAINING PRINCIPLES

Training Adaptations

Training adaptations are how the body responds to applied training stimulus throughout time. These adaptations can be either positive or negative depending on the type, volume, and intensity of the training stimulus. The goal of proper training is to manipulate these three factors to elicit a physiological response that will lead to positive training adaptations and increased performance. Incorrectly manipulating these factors can lead to negative adaptations and subsequent decreases in performance.

Individual Differences

The principle of individual differences states that not every individual will respond to the same training stimulus in the same manner. For example, some individuals recover quicker and can handle a higher training volume or intensity. Others may require longer recovery periods and therefore cannot handle higher volumes or frequent high-intensity bouts. You will need to individualize your training program so that you optimize training volume and recovery time.

While most individuals are born with approximately 50 percent slow-twitch muscle fibers (good for endurance) and 50 percent fast-twitch muscle fibers (good for anaerobic exercise, power, and strength), some individuals are born with a greater percentage of slow-twitch or fast-twitch fibers; therefore, some individuals will be predisposed to greater improvements in endurance, while others will be predisposed to greater improvements in anaerobic exercise, power, and strength. Fighters who have predominantly slow-twitch fibers tend to rely on the endurance, and those who have predominantly fast-twitch fibers tend to rely on their strength and power.

Current training status is also an obvious factor. Those who have been training longer will be able to handle greater volume and intensity in relation to beginners. Beginners will need to start by building a strong base and should avoid jumping into a training program designed for professional fighters.

Athletes and coaches often overlook individual differences and use a generic boxed training program that does not vary based on individual progression and can often hinder development. Too little stimulus can result in little to no improvement in a fighter's performance. Conversely, if the training program is too strenuous, it can lead to overtraining and burnout. That said, it is okay to use a boxed training program to begin with. When using a boxed training program, adjustments to volume and intensity should be made based on your response to that program.

Progressive Overload

The progressive overload principle states that the training stimulus needs to be continuously increased, allowing for adequate recovery between bouts, so that—ultimately—performance increases. You can increase stimulus by either increasing volume or intensity. Volume will be expressed as your overall training hours per week. Intensity is determined by how hard the workout session is conducted. Volume should always be increased prior to increasing intensity. Increasing intensity prior to increasing volume also increases the risk of injury.

As a mixed martial artist, it is important to monitor both training volume and intensity. You will be conducting martial arts training, as well as strength and conditioning training. Finding the appropriate mixture of training and recovery can be somewhat complicated.

While the overload principle is one of the key training principles, it must be used correctly. You cannot continuously increase stimulus and see gains. If you attempted this approach you would end up severely overtrained. Instead, you will need to undulate your program using periodization (discussed later in this book) so that you allow for periods of decreased volume and intensity for recovery and then ramp back up to higher volumes and intensities.

Principle of Hard and Easy

The hard–easy principle states that you cannot train hard every day and instead must alternate hard and easy days to optimize training adaptations. While this principle does oversimplify the problem, it does work, especially in the development of a training program for the beginning mixed martial artist. When designing a workout program, it is important to alternate your hard and easy days so that you will have ample time for recovery. Too many hard days in a row will result in overtraining due to lack of recovery between bouts. Examining intensity is one way to determine your hard and easy days. Sparring sessions, anaerobic sessions, plyometric sessions, or interval sessions are examples of hard days, whereas technique training or a recovery run would be considered easy days. Keep in mind that many times coaches intermix technique with anaerobic training, which would make it a hard day.

Recovery

Too often martial artists focus all of their energy on training and ignore one of the most important components of increasing performance: recovery. Training is catabolic (molecules are broken down into smaller constituents) in nature, ultimately resulting in protein synthesis after the training bout. To optimize the body's response to the training stimuli, you must make sure that adequate recovery occurs between bouts.

Alternating hard and easy days is a simple but effective way to optimize recovery. It is important to monitor intensity so that you do not train too hard too often. This is a common mistake made by most beginning fighters. Nutrition is an important component of recovery; therefore, it is vital to focus on recovery nutrition to refuel and optimize protein synthesis. Sleep is another component of recovery that is often overlooked. It is important that you maintain a minimum of eight hours of good sleep every night.

Tracking your morning heart rate is an excellent method for determining if you are recovered enough for that day's training. The simplest method is to measure heart rate with a heart rate monitor first thing in the morning while still in bed. After your alarm goes off, put on the heart rate monitor transmitter, lay back in bed, and relax as you monitor your heart rate. Record the lowest number displayed. Small deviations in heart rate are normal from day to day; however, if you have a significant increase in heart rate during the span of a couple days, you are overtrained. For example, if your morning resting heart rate is typically anchored at about 45 beats per minute (bpm) and you have a heart rate of 52 one day and 55 the next, chances are you are overtraining. Fluctuations in morning heart rate plus or minus 2 to 3 bpm are normal during training. Use of heart rate variability provides a better assessment of recovery but requires a greater understanding and more sensitive equipment.

Overtraining

One of the most common threats to athletic performance is overtraining. In almost every case, a fighter will compete better 10 percent undertrained as opposed to 1 percent overtrained. To optimize performance, mixed martial artists continually walk the line of optimal performance and overtraining. Overtraining occurs when adequate recovery is not allowed between bouts and is often the result of a sudden increase in volume and/or intensity, or an accumulation of a small imbalance of recovery and training.

As a mixed martial artist, you need to be aware of how your body responds to training and know the signs and symptoms of overtraining. Common signs of overtraining include the following:

- Experiencing multiple sessions of decreased performance. One bad day does not necessarily indicate overtraining; however, multiple days of decreased performance is a strong indication of overtraining.
- Feeling constant fatigue
- Exhibiting poor attitude
- Dreading an upcoming training session more than normal
- Experiencing abnormal sleeping patterns
- Experiencing an increase in resting heart rate measured on multiple days. An increase on one day may indicate that you have not recovered from the previous day's workout or that you may be dehydrated; however, if the

increase in resting heart rate persists during a span of multiple days, it is a strong indicator of overtraining.

- Suffering consistent overuse injuries
- Experiencing chronic illness due to a lowered immune response
- Displaying abrupt changes in body composition

Specificity of Training

Training adaptations are specific to the training stimulus applied. In simpler terms, train the body in the manner in which you would like for it to adapt. MMA requires that a fighter maintain an aerobic base and be capable of handling repeated anaerobic bouts. Muscular strength, muscular endurance, muscular power, and flexibility are also important components of MMA. This book provides information on how to create a program that allows you to optimally train in these areas. It is important to keep in mind that you are not training to be a bodybuilder, powerlifter, or endurance runner. It would make no sense to train and condition like a bodybuilder to compete as a mixed martial artist. Instead, you should incorporate all of these components into your program to optimize your performance.

Detraining

Detraining occurs when you decrease or remove the training stimulus, which leads to a decrease in performance and loss of training adaptations. Put quite simply, if you do not use it, you lose it. Common reasons for detraining include injury, illness, and improper offseason training. Typically, detraining begins after two weeks of inactivity. This does not mean that you lose all adaptations after two weeks of detraining. It just means that there is a measurable difference after two weeks of no training.

Detraining is one of the biggest fears of most fighters, which often leads to overtraining. Many mixed martial artists believe that taking a few days off from training will negatively impact performance, but taking a couple of days off on occasion will not hurt your performance and could, in fact, be beneficial if you are overtrained. Nevertheless, do not use the fear of overtraining as an excuse to take multiple days off on a regular basis. It is important to measure training progress to adequately determine if overtraining is occurring.

If you have to scale down or completely stop training due to illness or injury, it will not take too long to get back to where you left off. When returning to training, do not try to start at the same volume and intensity where you left off. Instead, start back up slowly and work your way back to the level at which you were training prior to your layoff. Focus on fighting technique, and slowly start increasing volume and then intensity. Coming back too quickly can lead to injury and further delays in training. This is especially true if the time off from training occurred due to injury.

Consistency

Your training plan should be well laid out and consistent in terms of frequency of training. One of the common mistakes beginners make is to train haphazardly—four days a week for a couple of weeks, then two days the following week, and then one day a week for the next couple of weeks. Increases in performance will be minimal at best.

Inconsistent training may also lead to injury. Trying to automatically pick up where you left off places too much stress on the body. For the best gains and to reduce the risk of injury, follow your training program. If life gets in the way, which it does, alter your training program to minimize the impact.

Frequency

Frequency is defined as how often you train. This can be measured in days or number of training sessions. Beginning mixed martial artists should train a minimum of three to five days per week, with a day off or easy day between workouts. This method allows you to train harder on workout days and then recover prior to your next workout.

To determine frequency of your workouts, first consider your current fitness level. As a beginner, you should start on the lower end and work your way up. The second thing to consider is the type of workout you have scheduled in your training plan. With MMA, you have technique training, sparring sessions, aerobic training, strength training, and anaerobic training, all of which you will need to incorporate into your training plan. This factor makes training for MMA more complicated in relation to other sports. There will be times when you will need to have two training sessions in one day, which requires careful planning to prevent overtraining.

Time management is an important skill to acquire if you plan on taking your training seriously. Other commitments, for example, family, work, and school, have to be considered when developing a training schedule. You need to find a way to balance every aspect of your life so that you are ultimately happy. For me, family will always come first, then work, then training.

Duration

Duration is the length of your training session, which will be determined by the goal of that session. Most often the duration of a session will be determined by the desired intensity. Duration and intensity are inversely related, meaning as one goes up the other must go down. The type of training that you are conducting can also impact the duration of a training session. Technique training conducted at a lower intensity can last longer than a session of interval training. This is why you always consider the duration and intensity of a training session. It is important to log your duration so that you can track your overall training volume.

Intensity

Intensity is the "how hard" of training, and it is extremely important to properly manipulate intensity for appropriate training adaptations to occur. The hard–easy principle is one method of manipulating training intensity. The hard–easy principle states that you cannot train hard every day and instead must alternate hard and easy days to optimize training adaptations. While this principle does oversimplify the problem, it does work, especially in the development of a training program for the beginner. Later in this book I discuss how to schedule your training to optimize this principle.

Intensity levels can be categorized into three basic levels: below anaerobic threshold, at anaerobic threshold, and above anaerobic threshold. An MMA fight is aerobic in nature with many anaerobic bouts. On average, the high intensity to low intensity ratio is 1:3 (meaning that you have one high intensity action for every three low intensity actions) during the average MMA fight. Knowing and understanding intensity levels allows you to better plan a training regimen to ensure that you do not overtrain.

Also keep in mind that how "hard" a training session is on the body will also be determined by the type of training you are conducting. An hour of sparring is hard on the body but so too is a session of plyometric training. So, having an understanding of what constitutes a hard session and what signifies an easy session becomes extremely important. To appropriately stress the body and allow adequate time for recovery, you must alternate hard and easy days.

A few examples of hard training sessions are as follows:

- Sparring session
- Any anaerobic session

- Plyometric training
- Strength-training session
- Long aerobic session (e.g., a long run)

A few examples of easy training sessions include the following:

- Technique sessions (ground, standing, MMA)
- Easy aerobic sessions (low in intensity and short in duration)
- Flexibility training
- Complete day of rest (yes, you need those)

Warm-ups

It is important to warm up prior to exercise to optimize performance and decrease the risk of injury. While a direct link between warming up and a decreased risk of injury has yet to be determined, there is a strong correlation between injury rates and lack of warming up. In regard to sport performance, warming up facilitates three important aspects. First, the warm-up will redirect blood flow to working muscles. Second, there will be an increase in cardiac output due to an increase in both heart rate and stroke volume. Third, muscle temperature will increase, which improves muscular performance. It typically takes about two minutes to sufficiently increase cardiac output, increase muscle temperature, and redirect blood flow to the point that oxygen supply is equivalent to demand in the working muscles. All of these factors will result in increased performance.

A warm-up for MMA should consist of about 10 minutes of easy cardio, for instance, jumping rope or jogging. Follow the cardio warm-up with about 5 to 10 minutes of stretching. For competition, the stretching should be primarily dynamic, and for training sessions, stretching should be an equal combination of static and dynamic. After stretching, finish off with skill-based warm-ups. Skill-based warm-ups consist of shadowboxing, pad work, light technique sparring, and other skill-based warm-up drills.

Your warm-up should end just prior to the start of training or competition. Do not exceed more than 5 to 10 minutes before the start of your next activity. If you end your warm-up more than 10 minutes before the start of the competition or training, you will begin to lose the benefits of the warm-up. The further out you stop, the more benefits you will lose.

Cooldown

Conducting a cooldown after a workout is an important part of your training program. An active cooldown will slowly bring your heart rate down and prevent blood from pooling in your legs. If you suddenly stop after a hard bout of exercise and blood pools in your legs, it could result in dizziness. While dizziness in these conditions is not overly common, it is not uncommon. As you continue to move during your active recovery, the muscle pump in the legs will assist with blood return to the heart and prevent blood from pooling in the legs. An active cooldown will also help clear blood lactate after high-intensity bouts; however, a cooldown will not prevent the development of delayed onset of muscle soreness.

A cooldown should consist of 5 to 10 minutes of light jogging or walking, followed by dynamic stretching leading into static stretching. The harder the workout, the longer the cooldown should be.

Delayed Onset of Muscle Soreness

If you work out it is inevitable that you will experience delayed onset of muscle soreness (DOMS). DOMS is the pain that you feel the day after a workout. This pain will typically last one to three days, depending on the extent of the muscular damage. In severe cases, DOMS can last much longer. There is a common misconception that DOMS occurs due to a buildup of lactic acid, but this is not the case. DOMS occurs due to tiny tears in muscle tissue that occur during eccentric contractions (muscle lengthens during the contraction). Edema occurs, and as the swelling continues it begins to push on nerve endings, resulting in pain.

BASIC PHYSIOLOGY

Physiology Overview

To correctly apply training principles to optimize performance it is important to have a basic understanding of physiology as it applies to sport performance. This understanding will allow you to determine the type of training stimulus that will best lead to adaptations for increased performance for MMA. There are many "experts" who claim to have the best method for increased performance. Too often these methods are unsubstantiated fads that will not lead to increased performance and, in some cases, lead to a decrease in performance. Because of this it is important that you are able to determine what will and will not work for you based on scientific evidence. The more educated you are on the subject, the better you will be able to make an informed decision.

Knowledge of physiology as it applies to MMA performance will help you better understand how to effectively develop a strong training program. If you understand how the body responds to exercise, it will allow you to use physiological markers to monitor training session intensity and recovery between sessions. An understanding of basic physiology as it applies to training will also allow you to determine if your body is correctly adapting to the applied training stimulus. If you understand the physiological adaptations that should occur, you can better gauge the degree to which your training program elicits these changes.

The key to understanding physiology is a term that was driven into my head throughout eight years of school (undergrad through Ph.D., not eight years of undergrad): form and function. Every element of the body is formed to perform a specific function. Adaptations occurring due to training may even slightly alter form to improve function. Understanding the function of a system, organ, hormone, substrate, or enzyme will allow you to determine the effect of each on human performance. This section covers basic physiology, which will build a strong foundation of knowledge that will allow you to better grasp the acute physiological responses to training, as well as the physiological adaptations that occur due to training. Understanding how the body functions will allow you to better determine your training and ultimately make you a better fighter.

Cardiorespiratory System

The cardiorespiratory system is comprised of the cardiovascular system and the respiratory system. The cardiovascular system is made up of the heart and blood vessels, and is responsible for the movement of blood throughout the body. Movement of blood throughout the body is responsible for transporting oxygen, glucose, free fatty acids, hormones, and other key substrates to the working muscle. Equally important are the byproducts that blood carries away from the working tissue (carbon dioxide, lactate, etc.).

The respiratory system is comprised of air passages and lungs, and is responsible for the transport and diffusion of gasses. Air moves through the air passageways, bringing in vital oxygen to the lungs, where it is diffused across the respiratory membrane and into blood. Carbon dioxide will diffuse from the blood, across the respiratory membrane, and into the lungs, where it is exhaled into the atmosphere.

The cardiorespiratory system is key during endurance performance and many times will limit performance based on the individual's current fitness level. Too often, fighters will "gas out" due to an insufficiently developed cardiorespiratory system. Adaptations that occur due to endurance training greatly improve the body's ability to transport blood and oxygen. These adaptations are discussed later in this chapter.

Heart

The heart is a specialized muscle (myocardium) designed to pump blood throughout the body. The heart differs from skeletal muscle in the following ways: It is the most oxidative muscle in the body, it is designed to rapidly conduct the electrical impulse, and the signal for contraction originates in the muscle (sinoatrial node) and therefore is involuntary. The heart consists of four chambers (left and right atria, and left and right ventricles). Pulmonary circulation (right atrium and ventricle) is designed to pump oxygen-poor blood returning from the body into the lungs. Systemic circulation (left atrium and ventricle) is designed to pump oxygen-rich blood to the body.

Oxygen-poor blood returns to the right side of the heart and then is pumped to the lungs, where CO_2 is released from the blood and O_2 is picked up. The oxygen-rich blood then travels to the left side of the heart, where it is pumped out to the body. The blood then travels through smaller and smaller arteries until it reaches arterioles and then capillaries at the tissue. This is where oxygen, nutrients, water, carbon dioxide, and other byproducts are transported to and from the tissue. As the capillaries leave the tissue, they connect to venules and then veins before returning to the heart.

The heart is not strong enough to pump blood throughout the body and then back toward the heart, against gravity from the lower extremities. There are mechanisms in place that assist with blood return to the heart. The first is called the muscle pump. Muscles in the leg contract rhythmically, causing blood to be pushed upward during the contraction phase. When the muscles relax, one-way valves in the veins prevent the blood from flowing back down. The second method is the respiratory pump. Changes in thoracic pressure due to breathing aid in blood return to the heart.

Cardiac Output

Cardiac output (Q) is the volume of blood pumped per minute. It is a product of stroke volume (SV) and heart rate (HR) ($Q = SV \times HR$). Stroke volume is the volume of blood pumped from the left ventricle each beat, and heart rate is defined as the number of times the heart beats each minute. Cardiac output responds to exercise by increasing linearly with increases in intensity until max intensity is reached. Heart rate also increases linearly with an increase in intensity. Stroke volume can almost double from resting, but it will only increase to about 50 percent of maximal intensity and then it levels off. So, after about 50 percent of maximal intensity, increases in cardiac output will come primarily from increases in heart rate only.

Autoregulation of Blood Flow

Autoregulation of blood flow concerns the redirection of blood flow based on tissue need. Blood flow is redirected by altering blood vessel diameter through vasoconstriction and vasodilatation. As you move from a resting state to an exercising state, metabolism substantially increases. Going for an easy run can increase metabolism by six to nine times above resting levels. Because the metabolic demand of the working muscles has increased substantially, a greater amount of blood flow must be sent to the working muscle to increase the delivery of oxygen and nutrients. During exercise, blood flow is redirected to the working muscles, skin (for cooling), heart, and brain. Blood flow is reduced in areas where less is needed, for instance, the digestive system and kidneys. During rest, approximately 20 percent of blood flow travels to the muscles. During exercise, as much as 80 percent of blood flow can be redirected to muscle.

Understanding this concept is vital in having a complete understanding of the body's response to exercise. For example, autoregulation of blood flow explains why warming up prior to training or competition is so important. As soon as you start exercising, metabolic demand increases immediately; however, it takes about two minutes to warm up and adequately redirect blood flow to the working muscles so that oxygen supply is equal to the demand. Warming up allows for the redirection of blood flow to the working muscles and other areas of need so that you begin your training session or competition ready to perform.

Due to autoregulation of blood flow the timing of meals also becomes important. Eating a meal too close to training or competition can result in gastrointestinal distress and subpar performance. This response is due to the digestive system being in direct competition with the working muscles for blood flow. Due to fight or flight, the sympathetic response will win out against the parasympathetic response, and greater blood flow will go to the muscles; however, in relation to exercising without prior food consumption, a greater amount of blood will be redirected to the digestive system for digestion. Because of the redirection of blood flow to the digestive system, there will be a decrease in performance and some level of gastrointestinal distress.

During exercise, internal heat production increases substantially due to the increase in metabolism. To maintain a safe core temperature, blood flow is increased to the skin for cooling. When exercising in the heat, a greater amount of blood flow will be redirected to the skin for cooling in relation to training in a thermoneutral environment. Dissipating heat is vital for survival and will take priority over blood flow to muscles. Due to this phenomenon, there will be a significant decrease in performance when training in a hot environment.

Blood

Blood is made up of about 55 percent plasma, 45 percent red blood cells (erythrocytes), and less than 1 percent white blood cells (leukocytes) and platelets. Hematocrit is used to measure the particular makeup of an individual's blood and defined as the ratio of red blood cells in relation to whole blood. The average hematocrit for a male is approximately 45, and for a female it is about 42.

Blood has five major roles: transportation, heat transfer, acid–base balance, coagulation, and immune response. While all five are important, we typically concentrate on the first three in exercise physiology, as they have the greatest impact on performance. Each red blood cell contains multiple hemoglobin molecules, which are responsible for the transportation of oxygen. Hemoglobin is comprised of a globin protein and a heme ring. The heme ring contains four iron molecules, and each of these iron molecules can bind one oxygen molecule. This is why those who suffer from iron deficiency feel fatigued and have difficulty exercising.

Blood is extremely important when it comes to heat dissipation. Water makes up about 90 percent of plasma, which is why plasma is an excellent mechanism for heat transfer. Heat is transferred from the core and working muscles to the blood, where it is dissipated at the skin surface. Plasma is also important for cooling, as it provides sweat for evaporation at the skin; this statement is oversimplified, as plasma moving from the blood vessels to the interstitial space to the skin is a complicated process.

It is vital that the acid–base balance is maintained for the body to correctly function. Keep in mind that pH differs depending on the location in the body. The average muscle pH is about 7.1, whereas the pH in the blood is about 7.4. A decrease in pH (increase in acidity) occurs during high-intensity exercise. It does not take a large drop in pH before physiological systems are affected. A drop in muscle pH from 7.1 to 6.9 will begin to negatively impact energy systems, leading to a decrease in performance. Blood helps maintain pH through the use of chemical buffers.

Gas Exchange

The main driving force for gas exchange in the body is the partial pressure of each gas. To understand the importance of partial pressure let's review Dalton's law: The sum of each individual pressure of each individual gas is equivalent to the total pressure of the mixture of gases. At sea level, the atmospheric pressure is equivalent to 760 millimeters of mercury (mmHg), which gives you the total pressure of the mixture of gases (air). What becomes important for understanding gas exchange is the partial pressure of each individual gas in the mixture. Oxygen makes up 20.93 percent of the total mixture, resulting in a partial pressure of oxygen (PO_2) equal to 159 mmHg. Carbon dioxide makes up .03 percent of the total mixture, resulting in a partial pressure of carbon dioxide (PCO_2) of .2 mmHg. Lastly, nitrogen accounts for 79.04 percent of the total mixture, resulting in a partial pressure of nitrogen (PN_2) of 600.7 mmHg.

One thing to keep in mind is that atmospheric pressure alters as you increase altitude from sea level. If you were to leave sea level and travel to the top of Mt. Evans in Colorado, the atmospheric pressure would decrease to approximately 460 mmHg. Because the atmospheric pressure decreases and there are no alterations to the percent of each individual gas, the partial pressure of each gas will decrease. If you live, train, or compete at altitude, this is an important concept to understand.

The alveoli are air sacs located at the end of air tubes located in the lungs, which are responsible for oxygen and carbon dioxide exchange. Gas exchange occurs across the respiratory membrane, which lies between the alveoli and capillaries. While the PO_2 in the atmosphere at sea level is equivalent to 159 mmHg, the PO_2 will decrease to about 105 mmHg in the lungs. At rest, oxygen-poor blood will return to the lungs at a PO_2 of about 40 mmHg. The pressure differential of 60 mmHg will cause oxygen to move from the alveoli to the capillaries. Because alveolar PO_2 is maintained at 105 mmHg (it is not a closed system), oxygenated blood will leave the heart at a PO_2 of approximately 100 mmHg.

The alveoli PCO_2 remains at a constant 40 mmHg. The PCO_2 of blood returning to the heart will be approximately 46 mmHg. While the pressure differential is not as large in relation to oxygen, carbon dioxide diffuses at a much greater rate across the respiratory membrane in relation to oxygen; therefore, the gradient does not have to be as large.

Muscle

Skeletal muscle originates and inserts on bone and will cross at least one joint; therefore, the primary purpose of skeletal muscle is human movement. There are more than 600 muscles in the human body, and it is important that you be able to name and identify all of them (just kidding). It is important that you learn the primary muscles used in MMA to ensure proper strengthening and flexibility of those muscles.

Each skeletal muscle is composed of numerous muscle fibers. These muscle fibers are classified by characteristics and divided into slow-twitch (type I) muscle fibers and fast-twitch (type II, with subcategories IIa and IIx, and recently discovered IIb) muscle fibers. Slow-twitch fibers are highly oxidative and resistant to fatigue, and therefore are optimal for endurance performance. Type II fibers are more glycolytic and produce more force, and therefore they are good for events that require anaerobic energetics, strength, and power.

Distribution of muscle fiber type is genetic; most people are born with 50 percent slow-twitch fibers and 50 percent fast-twitch fibers. Some individuals are born with a greater amount of one type of fiber or another. Elite-level endurance athletes will typically possess as much as 80 percent slow-twitch fibers, whereas an elite-level Olympic lifter can have as much as 65 percent fast-twitch fibers. The predominate theory is that muscle fiber types cannot change from one type to another through training. Muscle fiber distribution can be determined through a muscle biopsy, which is expensive and painful, and therefore typically not recommended.

For MMA, distribution of fiber type will affect your overall strategy when fighting. Lighter fighters will most likely have a higher percentage of slow-twitch fibers and therefore have greater endurance and less power, whereas many heavier fighters will have a greater volume of fast-twitch fibers. For this reason, lighter fighters are able to sustain higher outputs for longer durations during a fight and can recover quicker between rounds. Conversely, heavier fighters can throw strikes with greater power but will fatigue much quicker.

Muscle fibers are arranged in functional groups called motor units. Each motor unit consists of only one type of muscle fiber and is innervated by a motor neuron. A slow-twitch motor unit will have a small amount of muscle fibers, whereas a fast-twitch motor unit will contain a much larger number of muscle fibers. The number of motor units in a muscle is highly dependent on the size of the muscle. The larger the muscle, the more motor units that muscle will contain.

It is important to understand how motor units function and how they are recruited to contract. When the signal to contract travels down the motor neuron to the muscle fibers of the motor unit, every muscle fiber in that unit will contract. This is known as the all-or-none response. It is like a light switch—it is either on or off. But not all of the motor units in a muscle will contract during a task. We recruit only the exact number of motor units necessary to accomplish the task at hand.

Motor units are recruited in a specific pattern based on the size of the motor unit. Due to this, slow-twitch motor units are recruited first, followed by fast-twitch fibers. Recruitment is designed for optimal economy. The higher the intensity, the greater the amount of fast-twitch fibers that will be recruited. As fast-twitch fibers are not very oxidative, you will fatigue sooner at higher intensities.

Through training, neuromuscular recruitment patterns are altered, allowing you to become more proficient at the skill. Neuromuscular recruitment patterns deal with the timing and force of the muscle recruited to conduct a specific skill, for instance, a Thai kick. As you continue to practice, the neuromuscular recruitment patterns will improve to perform the skill in the manner in which you train the skill. This adaptation improves economy and ultimately performance. This is why it is important to work skill training over and over until you adopt the correct neuromuscular recruitment patterns. An incorrect neuromuscular recruitment pattern will be hard to alter once developed.

Energy Systems

Energy is required for human movement to occur. Competing in MMA requires repetitive muscle contractions and significant increases in metabolism. As you move from resting to exercise, metabolism increases exponentially. Going from resting metabolism to just a jog increases energy requirements six to nine times that of resting requirements.

There are three primary sources for energy: lipids, carbohydrates, and proteins. Of the three sources, lipids and carbohydrates provide the vast majority of energy during exercise. With the exception of extreme situations (starvation or a no-carb diet), protein will never provide a substantial source of energy. The main job of protein involves anabolic processes in the body. Carbohydrates are stored as glycogen in the muscles and liver, and transported in the blood as glucose. Glycogen stored are limited to approximately 2,000 kilocalories (kCals). Lipids are stored as triacylglycerol (commonly referred to as triglycerides) in muscle and adipose tissue (under the skin and around organs). Storage of lipids varies greatly among individuals, with the average being 60,000 to 80,000 kCals. Excess protein is not stored in the body. Regardless of the source, all ingested food must be converted to adenosine triphosphate (ATP) to be used as fuel in the human body.

Energy systems are frequently categorized into aerobic and anaerobic systems. Aerobic systems are those systems that require oxygen for the metabolic processes to occur, and anaerobic systems are those that do not require oxygen for metabolic processes to occur. In each of those broad categories (aerobic and anaerobic) there are four basic energy systems that provide ATP for human movement. It is important to understand each of these energy systems because they impact training, competition, and choice of nutrition.

Stored ATP

The first system is stored ATP in the muscles. While commonly classified as a system, stored ATP is more of a source as opposed to an actual system. Stores are limited; therefore, reliance on this system as a major energy source is also limited. Stored ATP will only provide energy for about two to three seconds before stores are depleted. Energy for the muscle contraction is provided when a phosphate is cleaved from ATP, leaving adenosine diphosphate (ADP) and a phosphate. This process does not require oxygen and provides energy fast for immediate contraction. The remaining three energy systems are methods of producing ATP for energy. Once ATP is generated through these systems, a phosphate must be cleaved off to release the energy for muscle contraction.

ATP-PC$_r$ System

The second system is the ATP-PC$_r$ system. Phosphocreatine (PC$_r$) is stored in the muscle and is key in producing ATP. During this process, a phosphate is cleaved from PC$_r$ and donated to an ADP to form ATP. The ATP-PC$_r$ system is limited by PC$_r$ stores in the muscle and can only function as a major energy system for about 10 to 15 seconds. This system is anaerobic in nature and does not require oxygen to function. It takes about two minutes of recovery for PC$_r$ stores to replenish. This is a key consideration when planning rest intervals during resistance training.

Anaerobic Glycolysis

The next energy system is anaerobic glycolysis, which provides ATP through the catabolism of glucose and glycogen. This process does not require oxygen and can provide energy for as much as a minute and a half to two minutes.

Anaerobic glycolysis produces two to three ATP per glucose or glycogen molecule. A decrease in pH is the limiting factor for energy production during anaerobic glycolysis. Muscle pH will decrease due to the hydrogen buildup that occurs during glycolysis. Glycolysis is a complex chemical process that stops at the creation of pyruvate. During anaerobic glycolysis, two hydrogen bind with pyruvate to form lactic acid, which in turn will lose one hydrogen, becoming lactate. Lactic acid production is based on intensity level, which determines the speed of glycolysis and oxygen availability for metabolism.

Lactic acid is often considered bad; however, this assumption is not correct, as lactic acid is formed to decrease acidity. As mentioned earlier, pyruvate picks up the excess hydrogen to decrease acidity. This binding is only temporary, and lactic acid releases the hydrogen ions and is converted into lactate (a salt molecule). Lactic acid itself is not the problem; instead, it is the buildup of hydrogen. Hydrogen ions greatly increase acidity and will interfere with muscle contraction. The pain felt during high-intensity exercise, for example, intervals, is the body's mechanism to signal you to slow down or come to a stop. Upon completion of exercise, lactic acid is converted back into fuel through specific pathways and therefore should not be considered a waste product.

Lastly, lactic acid is not responsible for DOMS. Delayed onset of muscle soreness is the soreness felt the day after a workout that can last one or more days depending on the damage done during exercise. DOMS is not caused by lactic acid, but instead by tiny tears in muscle tissue that occur during eccentric contractions.

Oxidative Phosphorylation

The first three systems provide energy quickly and without oxygen. The last system is oxidative phosphorylation, which will be used as the primary energy system for activity lasting longer than two minutes. Oxidative phosphorylation, as the name suggests, relies on oxygen for ATP production. There are two major pathways for energy production that fall under oxidative phosphorylation: the oxidation of carbohydrates and the oxidation of lipids. Duration and intensity will determine reliance on carbohydrates and lipids. Longer duration and lower intensity training will rely heavily on the oxidation of lipids, and high-intensity training that is shorter in duration will rely more heavily on the oxidation of carbohydrates.

The first pathway in oxidative phosphorylation is the oxidation of carbohydrates, which produces ATP through the catabolism of glucose and glycogen. This process is often termed *aerobic glycolysis*. The steps in aerobic glycolysis are the exact same as those in anaerobic glycolysis. The main difference is that instead of pyruvate being converted to lactic acid, it is converted to acetyl-CoA, which moves on to the Krebs cycle (citric acid cycle) for ATP production. Aerobic glycolysis produces 36 to 39 ATP from one molecule of glucose or glycogen. The limiting factor for oxidation of carbohydrates is the amount of stored glycogen. As previously mentioned, the average stores of glycogen are equivalent to about 2,000 kCals. Limited glycogen stores will not be a factor during an MMA competition. Limited glycogen stores start becoming an issue during continuous exercise lasting longer than an hour and a half.

The second pathway in oxidative phosphorylation involves the oxidation of lipids. This process requires more oxygen, more chemical processes, and more time; however, ATP production is much greater with the oxidation of lipids. One triacylglycerol will produce approximately 460 ATP. With 60,000 to 80,000 kCals of lipids stored in the body, it would be impossible to completely deplete during exercise. When fatigue occurs due to limitations of oxidative phosphorylation, it occurs due to depletion of glycogen stores, as you need glycogen to completely break down lipids.

VO_2 MAX

MMA is an endurance sport with numerous anaerobic bouts. There is a strong correlation between an athlete's oxidative capacity and their ability to maintain a high level of output throughout an entire fight, and how quickly they can recover between rounds. Because of this, it has become common practice to test a fighter's VO_2 max to determine current aerobic fitness level. VO_2 max is the body's maximal ability to deliver oxygen to the working muscles and the muscles' ability to use that oxygen to produce energy for movement. As VO_2 max increases with training, so too will cardiorespiratory endurance.

VO_2 max can be increased through aerobic training. The adaptations that occur due to endurance training are designed to increase oxygen transport and utilization. So, as aerobic training increases, VO_2 max increases, and so too does performance. The extent to which VO_2 max can be increased through training is highly dependent on genetics. While everyone can increase VO_2 max, improvements are limited by a predetermined genetic ceiling.

VO_2 max can be expressed in absolute (l/m) or relative terms (ml/kg/min). Expressing VO_2 max through relative terms is the preferred method, as it more accurately represents endurance performance relative to body mass, milliliters of oxygen consumed per kilogram of body mass each minute. As there is a strong linear relationship between VO_2 max measures and endurance performance, it is often used to predict performance. While there are currently no established norms for VO_2 max measures for MMA fighters, an ideal number would be, at minimum, 55 ml/kg/min. One of the reasons that there are no current norms is that it will vary by weight class. Smaller fighters will most likely have higher percentages of slow-twitch fibers and therefore higher VO_2 max measures in relation to heavyweight fighters who have a higher percentage of fast-twitch fibers and therefore lower VO_2 max measures.

VO_2 max is measured during a graded exercise protocol conducted in a laboratory setting. Testing is typically conducted on a treadmill, where the graded exercise protocol starts easy and intensity increases at regular time intervals until complete exhaustion. Most protocols consist of two- or three-minute stages. Intensity increases during the treadmill protocol by increasing both speed and grade. During the graded exercise protocol, gas exchange of O_2 and CO_2 is measured using an automated metabolic cart. This requires the participant to wear an airtight mask that allows them to breathe in room air and breathe out into a gas-mixing chamber. From the gas-mixing chamber, the air is analyzed for O_2 and CO_2.

Measurement of VO_2 max requires expensive, specialized equipment and trained personnel to run the test and evaluate the data. As such, testing is typically expensive. Testing will typically run between \$100 and \$300 depending on the facilities, testing personnel, and other services offered. Testing can be conducted at local performance centers and universities. The best option would be to contact the exercise physiology (kinesiology, physical education, or exercise science) department at your local university. Most researchers are always looking for subjects and will offer low-cost or free testing.

ANAEROBIC THRESHOLD/LACTATE THRESHOLD

Threshold terminology is used a lot in sports performance, but few people actually understand or know how to correctly apply the concept. The two most common terms used are *anaerobic threshold* and *lactate threshold*. Anaerobic threshold is defined as the point at which metabolic processes begin to switch from aerobic energetics to anaerobic energetics. Lactate threshold is defined as the point at which lactate production exceeds the body's ability to remove it. You are always producing lactate, even at rest, but it is removed from the system before it begins to build up. As intensity increases during exercise, lactate production increases, and there will come a point where production will exceed removal. As intensity increases, reliance on glycogen as a fuel source increases to the point that hydrogen is being produced at such a rate that it begins to build up, leading to a decrease in pH. To offset this decrease in pH, two hydrogen will bind with pyruvate to form lactic acid. This is unstable, and a hydrogen is released, forming lactate.

There are two common methods for measuring lactate threshold. The first method involves plotting blood lactate as intensity increases to determine the inflection point. The second method is referred to as onset of blood lactate accumulation, and it is marked at four millimoles per liter of blood. Using four millimoles per liter of blood is somewhat arbitrary and not overly accurate; therefore, it is typically not used to determine threshold. To obtain lactate threshold using either method, a graded exercise protocol would be conducted where resistance is systematically increased every three minutes until exhaustion. Blood would be taken at the end of every workload and analyzed for blood lactate.

A third method for determining anaerobic threshold is termed ventilator threshold (VT). This is the point at which ventilation increases exponentially and is easily calculated from data collected during a VO_2 max test. Ventilation increases as a direct response to the increased CO_2 production that occurs due to buffering excessive hydrogen. I typically prefer using VT to determine anaerobic threshold because it is accurate and easy, and I do not have to draw blood.

Regardless of the method used to determine anaerobic threshold, it will be expressed as either a percentage of max or relative to heart rate. An untrained individual can have an anaerobic threshold of about 70 percent of max, whereas an elite endurance athlete will have a threshold of approximately 90 percent of max. To use anaerobic threshold to monitor training intensity, you will need to know heart rate at anaerobic threshold.

TRAINING ADAPTATIONS

Adaptations to Endurance Training

Almost every adaptation that occurs due to endurance training is designed to increase the delivery of oxygen to the working muscles and increase the oxidative processes that occur within the working muscles. The entire point of your cardiorespiratory training program is to elicit these adaptations to improve performance. The purpose of this section is to identify the primary adaptations and explain the importance of each.

With endurance training there will be an increase in overall blood volume. Red blood cells will increase to boost the oxygen-carrying capacity of the blood.

Plasma volume will also increase but to a greater extent. Plasma increases for two primary reasons. The first is in response to the increased red blood cell volume. Plasma is the fluid portion of the blood responsible for the smooth transfer of the more viscous red blood cells. So, if there is an increase in red blood cells, there will be a corresponding increase in plasma. Plasma volume also increases in response to the heavy sweating and plasma loss, which occur during training. The increase in plasma volume will assist in heat dissipation and thermoregulation because there is a large increase in plasma volume in relation to the red blood cell increase. Hematocrit will decrease in trained individuals.

Increased blood volume would do no good if delivery at the muscles was not also increased. In response to the greater oxygen demand, capillary density will increase at the tissue, primarily the working muscles. The increased capillary density will supply more blood to the working muscles, allowing for greater gas, nutrient, and metabolic byproduct exchange.

Improved cardiac function also occurs as an adaptation to endurance training. As mentioned earlier, cardiac output equals stroke volume multiplied by heart rate (Q = SV x HR). With cardiorespiratory training, there will be an increase in stroke volume, which affects both cardiac output and heart rate. Stroke volume increases for three primary reasons. The first is that there will be a healthy enlargement of the left ventricle, allowing a greater volume of blood to enter. The increased blood volume will result in a larger volume of blood returning to the heart and therefore greater filling. Lastly, the cardiac muscle will produce a more forceful contraction. Because SV has increased, there will be a corresponding decrease in HR at any submaximal intensity, because cardiac output for that given submaximal intensity has not greatly altered. This is why resting heart rate will decrease as your cardiorespiratory fitness increases. Max heart rate does not alter with training and remains relatively constant. Due to the increase in stroke volume and no alteration in max HR, there will be an increase in maximum cardiac output with endurance training.

Alterations to muscle fiber will also occur with cardiorespiratory training. Type I muscle hypertrophy occurs, leading to improved performance. Type IIa (intermediate fibers) will shift toward oxidative properties. There will also be an increase in myoglobin to increase oxygen-carrying capacity within the muscle. Mitochondria (the oxidative powerhouse of the cell) will increase, leading to an increase in oxidative processes. There will be an overall increase in oxidative enzymes as well.

Changes to energy sources will also occur due to cardiorespiratory training. Three will be an increase in glycogen stores. Lipid stores will decrease in adipose tissue and increase in muscle. This will provide greater lipid stores in the muscles readily available for production of ATP. Lastly, you will begin to use fat at a higher percentage earlier during prolonged exercise to spare glycogen.

The last adaptation is an increase in lactate threshold, due to a decrease in lactic acid production and an increase in lactate clearance. While endurance training, especially tempo work, will increase lactate threshold, anaerobic training is key to increasing lactate threshold.

Adaptations to Anaerobic Training

Anaerobic training will result in various adaptations that will increase your anaerobic capacity, allowing you to maintain high-energy outputs for a longer period of time. One of the main adaptations that occurs due to anaerobic training involves an increase in anaerobic threshold due to an increased buffering capacity. As mentioned earlier, during high-intensity exercise, which relies on anaerobic glycolysis, hydrogen builds up in the system. This buildup of hydrogen results in a decrease in pH (increased acidity). There are two primary methods used to buffer this decrease in pH. The first is that two hydrogen will bind with pyruvate to form lactic acid, and the second is when sodium bicarbonate binds with hydrogen to form carbonic acid. When you increase your buffering capacity, you greatly increase the intensity at which you can compete, as well as the duration for which you can hold the intensity. The increase in anaerobic threshold also occurs because of an increase in glycolytic enzymes, which enhances energy production through glycolysis. There is also an increase in pain tolerance in individuals who train anaerobically. With a minimum of eight weeks of high-intensity training you can significantly increase your anaerobic threshold.

Another adaptation to anaerobic training is an increase in muscular strength. This adaptation correlates with the strongest increases in anaerobic performance. This concept has been reverse engineered by strength and conditioning coaches for years, with great effect. While these increases in strength from anaerobic training are great for improved performance alone, coaches have realized that implementing strength training and power training programs will in turn improve the athlete's anaerobic performance.

Anaerobic training will also improve motor unit recruitment and the stretch-shortening cycle, both of which will increase the ability of muscle to contract forcefully and quickly. This improvement occurs due to an increase in motor unit recruitment, an increase in the firing rate of the recruited motor units, and an improved stretch reflex response.

Adaptations to Resistance Training

When you begin a resistance training program you will see a large increase in the first eight weeks of training. Keep in mind that eight weeks is an average number that assumes you have not been active in resistance training. When someone new to resistance training begins a program, they will see somewhat steady gains for about the first eight weeks and then level off. This is because the first eight weeks of training result in neuromuscular adaptations that improve performance without a correlating increase in muscle fiber size (hypertrophy). These neuromuscular adaptations consist of increased motor unit recruitment, increased synchronization of motor unit and muscle activation, and a reduction in the golgi tendon organ (a sensory organ that limits force development as a protective mechanism) threshold.

After the first eight weeks of resistance training, you will begin to see increases in muscle fiber diameter (hypertrophy). To understand hypertrophy, you must first have an understanding of basic muscle structure. A muscle is made up of fasciculi bound together by connective tissue. Each individual fasciculus is made up of a bundle of muscle fiber, and each muscle fiber is made up of a bundle of myofibril. Within the myofibril you have actin and myosin, which work together to cause a contraction of the muscle. Hypertrophy occurs due to an increase in the number of actin and myosin within each myofibril and an increase in the number of myofibrils within each muscle fiber. To date, there is no strong evidence to support an increase in the number of muscle fibers within a muscle (hyperplasia) in humans.

PSYCHOLOGICAL TRAINING

We focus so much on the physiological and biomechanical principles of sport and often overlook the psychological factors of sport performance. Your psychological state can directly impact your physiological performance on many different levels. For example, your heart rate will increase in anticipation of a workout or competition without any increase in physical demand. The greater the anxiety, the higher your heart rate will be prior to participation. There is nothing wrong with an anticipatory increase in heart rate, and, as a matter of fact, starting your warm-up with a higher heart rate is beneficial. This section is not designed to give you an in-depth knowledge of sport psychology, but instead will hit on some key factors that will help with your performance.

Anxiety

Anxiety is a feeling of apprehension, nervousness, or fear that is in response to an event. While anxiety is a psychological construct, there is a corresponding physiological response. Anxiety results in increased activity of the sympathetic nervous system, leading to an increase in cardiac output, a redirection of blood flow, tightening of muscles, and gastrointestinal distress. It is quite common to feel anxious about an upcoming competition or event, and everyone experiences anxiety prior to a fight.

Being anxious is not entirely a bad thing, as it triggers your fight-or-flight response and prepares your body for the fight; however, it is not good to be overly anxious. Focusing on your anxiety prevents you from focusing on the fight at hand and can lead to negative physiological responses (tight muscles, gastrointestinal distress, etc.).

Attention/Focus

When training for and competing in MMA, it is important to focus on what your opponent is doing at all times. To accomplish this task, you must focus on their movements and ignore all other cues. The term *selective attention* is used to describe an athlete's focus on performance-relative cues while ignoring all nonessential cues. You have to block out all the commotion going on around you and in your own mind, and focus on the movement of your opponent. This skill takes a long time to master and does not come easily to many fighters.

Visualization

If you can visualize a movement or sequence of movements, it will greatly increase your ability to perform those movements. This theory holds true for anything from bench-pressing to striking combinations. Visualizing the movement in your head as you produce the movement allows you to better conduct the movement. To effectively use visualization, it is vital that you know and understand the appropriate sequencing of the techniques.

The ability to correctly use visualization is a learned process and takes time to master. Video recordings of performances can help the athlete with visualization. Oftentimes, with beginners, it is hard to visualize proper technique. The coach will explain to the athlete that they are conducting the technique incorrectly, but the athlete does not understand because they feel that they are doing the technique correctly. When the coach shows the athlete the video and details what they are doing incorrectly, the athlete can now better visualize what to change, as well as the correct technique.

Desensitization

Desensitization is the process by which you work to reduce the impact of a stimulus. It is a normal human reaction to close your eyes and flinch away from a punch or kick that is coming at your face. While normal, it is counterproductive to becoming a good fighter. You need to become desensitized to getting hit when sparring so that you flinch less and respond more appropriately, but this does not mean you should learn to take punches like Rocky Balboa.

To work on the desensitization process, simply get accustomed to getting hit. When working on this process it is important to go easy and work with a partner that has control. Start by hitting softly and then slightly increase as time goes by. Unless you plan on fighting, do not work up to hitting hard. Starting off your fighting experience by sparring hard may have a negative impact on this process and cause you to flinch even more.

Motivation

Motivation is the force that drives the way that you respond to situations. Motivation is not always simple and straightforward. Oftentimes motivation is multifaceted, complicated, and not always clear. Everyone reading this book will have different motivations for training in MMA. There are many reasons to become involved in MMA—for the competition, to get in shape, for self-defense, for military training, or for the simple love of combat arts. Most often, however, there is more than one factor that motivates someone to get involved. Taking the time to sit down and understand your motivation to train will allow you to better focus on your training plan and long-term goals.

Motivation can be either intrinsic (from within) or extrinsic (outside sources). Intrinsic motivation will have the largest impact on your performance in the long run, as the focus comes from your own desires. Intrinsic motivation is driven by your desire to excel, curiosity, love of the sport, desire to learn, desire to be challenged, and so on. As your desires are self-motivated, it is less likely that you will experience burnout or frequent changes in attitude toward training and competing. Intrinsic motivation leads to greater learning, focus, self-confidence, and satisfaction.

Extrinsic motivation can be either beneficial or harmful to performance. Examples of extrinsic motivation are monetary reward, trophies, external praise or lack thereof (from your coach, parents, friends, etc.), contracts, scholarships, and so forth. The problem with extrinsic motivation is that it is completely out of the athlete's control, and there is a danger that the athlete will focus their self-worth on these extrinsic factors. Extrinsic motivators can also lead to anxiety. Extrinsic motivators work best when the athlete has strong intrinsic motivation and the extrinsic motivation is not overemphasized. Moreover, those who focus solely on extrinsic motivators will burn out easier and not develop as quickly.

Setting Goals

When developing a program, it is important to establish both long-term and short-term goals to develop a long-range training plan. When working with a new athlete, I first want to know their long-term goals. This allows me to determine their overall motivation for training and build a successful program for them to reach those goals. It is difficult to develop a plan without knowing where you want to go.

Goals should be challenging, while remaining realistic and attainable. It is okay to set a high goal, for instance, becoming a professional fighter; however, it is not realistic to set the goal for your first year of training. For most people I would not recommend a competitive fight within their first year of training. It is always a good idea to talk over your goals with your coach so you can get them set and develop a plan.

To set your goals there are specific questions that you should ask yourself. They are as follows:

- Overall, what do I want to accomplish? Fitness? Self-defense? Competition? A combination of any of the three?
- What is my current fitness level?
- What is my current skill level?
- How much time can I dedicate to training?
- What are my logistical challenges?

These are examples of some of the basic questions you can ask yourself to help determine your goals. It is important to think about each question and answer as honestly as possible.

When setting goals, it is important to set both short-term and long-term goals. Look at it like a ladder. If you only had the bottom and top rungs of the ladder, it would be virtually useless, and you would be unable to climb to the top (your ultimate goal). Adding rungs (short-term goals) to the ladder between the bottom and top will allow you to climb easily and ultimately reach your goal. The journey to reach your ultimate goal can be difficult, long, and, at times, discouraging. Short-term goals give you something to strive for along the way.

After determining your short-term and long-term goals, write them down for future reference. The act of writing down your goals makes it much more likely that you will stick to those goals. Place your goals where you can see them daily so they will provide motivation along your journey.

Do Not Make Comparisons

One of the worst mistakes a fighter can make is to compare their progression with the skill level of other fighters. This is doubly true when a beginner attempts to compare their current level to an elite-level fighter. It is important to remember that the elite fighter started where you currently stand and progressed to an elite level through hard training and dedication. Do not focus on if you are better than someone else. Instead, focus on if you are better today than you were yesterday. If you ask yourself if you are better today than you were yesterday and the answer is "yes," you are going in the right direction. If the answer is "no," you need to evaluate your motivation, consistency, and training plan to determine why and make appropriate changes.

This concept does not mean that you should not realistically determine where your skill level is in relation to others if you plan to compete. Never compete before you are ready, as it can result in not only possible physical damage, but also psychological damage.

3

AREAS OF TRAINING FOR MIXED MARTIAL ARTS

A long with your technique training (Muay Thai, jiujitsu, boxing, etc.), you will need to work on strength and conditioning to optimize your performance. In this chapter I will define the primary areas of training and give example workouts for each area. For each type of training, there are more methods for working out than what is listed here. For example, there are different abdominal workouts that are not listed below. It does not mean that the other methods are not valid, I just chose a few movements to get you started. This book is not designed to be all inclusive, but to provide you a strong base on which you can build a solid program.

AEROBIC TRAINING

Aerobic training is designed to improve your cardiorespiratory endurance. As stated earlier, a fight is considered aerobic with anaerobic bouts. How often have you or someone you know "gassed out" early in a sparring round? This early fatigue occurs due to an insufficient aerobic base. Your aerobic base is important for not only maintaining the steady pace of the fight, but also recovery between rounds.

Naturally, a lot of your technique training will improve your cardiorespiratory endurance. While sparring rounds are an excellent way to improve your aerobic capacity, they will not provide enough of an adaptation to elevate your cardiorespiratory endurance to the level needed to optimize performance. You will need to add in aerobic training sessions on top of your technique training.

Type of Aerobic Training

The first thing you will need to decide is what type of aerobic training you would like to participate in. Unfortunately, the answer cannot be, "None! I do not want to participate in any!" The trick is to find something that you enjoy doing and effectively improves your aerobic capacity. The easiest type of cardiovascular training that you can participate in is running. It requires little equipment, is the least time consuming, and can be conducted just about anywhere; therefore, this book mainly focuses on running for aerobic training. While running is the easiest form of aerobic training, there are other options. Rowing is an excellent training method; it provides a full aerobic body workout that translates well to mixed martial arts (MMA).

Frequency of Training

Frequency for your endurance training should be approximately three to four days per week. Keep in mind that you must schedule your aerobic training so that it fits in with the rest of your training. The biggest danger to your training is trying to do too much. Oftentimes fighters will look at a runner's training program, which recommends running five to seven days a week, and then try to fit in that running program on top of the rest of their training schedule. You are not training to be a runner; you are training to be a fighter. The aerobic portion of your program is just one piece of the overall program and should be treated as such.

Intensity of Training

Determining the intensity of your aerobic training program is very important. One of the most accurate ways to determine intensity is by measuring heart rate. Heart rate is the number of times the heart beats per minute and can be measured using a heart rate monitor that detects the electrical impulse of the contractions. This method of determining heart rate makes it an easy and practical tool for determining intensity. You can also manually count pulse rate at the carotid or radial arteries, but this method is very inaccurate.

To use heart rate as a training tool, you need to determine your heart rate max, which is the maximal times your heart can beat in one minute measured at maximal intensity. Once heart rate max is determined, training zones can be determined based on a percentage of heart rate max.

To truly determine maximal heart rate, you have to push your body to maximal intensity. This is typically accomplished by conducting a VO_2 max testing protocol or hill repeats. A VO_2 max testing protocol is executed in a laboratory setting. The test protocol starts at an easy intensity and increases resistance every two to three minutes, depending on the protocol, until complete exhaustion. Aside from heart rate max, the testing protocol will provide information on your VO_2 max (a strong measure of endurance performance) and your heart rate at anaerobic threshold.

Another method for determining maximal heart rate is hill repeats. To conduct hill repeats, you will warm up and then perform multiple hill sprints until volitional exhaustion while wearing a heart rate monitor. Hill repeats do not provide as much information as a VO_2 max protocol; however, they are easy to execute, do not require special equipment, and will provide you with an accurate heart rate max.

Now that heart rate max has been established, you can determine intensity levels based on heart rate using training zones. Training zone heart rates will set the parameters of your training session by providing an upper and lower heart rate limit. During the training session, you want your heart rate to stay between the prescribed lower and upper limits. Most heart rate monitors will have training zone alarms that will alert you when you move out of your designated training zone for that particular session. There may be times when you have to go out of your training zone. For example, if you live in a hilly area and you have to run a steep hill on your route, that increases your heart rate above your upper limit even though you are running the hill as easily as possible.

There are many different recommended heart rate training zones, and, if applied correctly, most all of them work. I discuss the basic four-zone method in this book. As this section is focused on aerobic training, only zones 1 through 3 apply. Zone 4 is for anaerobic training, discussed later.

- Zone 1: Active Recovery
  - 50 to 65 percent of heart rate max
  - Training below 70 percent ensures that it is an active recovery day.
- Zone 2: Aerobic
  - 70 to 80 percent of heart rate max
  - For beginners, 80 percent may be too high, and you may want to consider staying closer to 70 percent.
  - This is where the majority of your training will occur.
- Zone 3: Threshold
  - 80 to 90 percent of heart rate max
  - This zone will typically fall into race pace or tempo training.

- Zone 4: Interval
  - 90 to 100 percent of max heart rate
  - This will be your high-intensity training above threshold.

You can also set heart rate training zones using heart rate at anaerobic threshold. You can only train at three physiological intensities: below threshold, at threshold, and above threshold. If you know the heart rate that corresponds to your current anaerobic threshold, you can set training zones based on that anchor point. As stated earlier, this section is focused on aerobic training, and only zones 1 through 3 apply. Zone 4 is for anaerobic training. The four zones when using threshold heart rate are as follows:

- Zone 1: Active Recovery
  - 25 percent or more below threshold heart rate
- Zone 2: Aerobic
  - 25 to 10 percent below threshold heart rate
- Zone 3: Threshold
  - ± 10 percent of threshold heart rate
- Zone 4: Interval
  - > 110 percent of heart rate threshold

While heart rate monitors are great training tools, you can also determine intensity based on feel. The talk test is easy to use and an effective tool for determining intensity. To keep it simple, the talk test will allow you to determine if you are below, at, or above threshold. If you are training below threshold, you should be able to hold a decent conversation. The closer you get to threshold, the harder it will be to hold a conversation. At threshold, you should only be able to get out a short sentence, at most. Above threshold, you may get out one word, at most. I found this to be an effective tool when working with beginners, especially when trying to keep them easy on an easy day. I simply told them that if they could not hold a conversation, slow down until they could at least get out two to three sentences.

Duration of Training

The next consideration is the duration of your aerobic training, which will vary based on the goal of that particular training session. Keep in mind that a full fight will be between 11 minutes (three 3-minute rounds with one minute of recovery between rounds) and 29 minutes (five 5-minute rounds with one minute of recovery between rounds). Your longest duration for aerobic training should be between 30 and 60 minutes. Keep in mind that you are not trying to be a runner. Instead, you are increasing your aerobic capacity to improve your fighting performance. There is a strong inverse relationship between intensity and duration. Your lower-intensity runs will be your longer runs, and your higher-intensity runs will be your shorter runs.

ANAEROBIC TRAINING

The terms *anaerobic power* and *capacity* are often used interchangeably. For simplicity, I will use the term *anaerobic power* during this section. Anaerobic power is the body's maximal ability to use anaerobic metabolic processes during high-intensity exercise: the ATP-PC$_r$ system and anaerobic glycolysis. MMA bouts require high and repeated anaerobic bouts. With just eight weeks of high-intensity training, you will see a large improvement in buffering capacity, which will allow you to increase your high-intensity efforts and recover quicker between high-intensity bouts.

Unlike aerobic capacity, there are no methods for directly measuring anaerobic power. Instead, tests are used to estimate anaerobic power. The Wingate test is the most common test used to estimate anaerobic power. The Wingate test is an all-out 30-second sprint on a stationary bike where the resistance is set at 7.5 percent of the athlete's body mass in kilograms. Peak and mean power are typically used to estimate anaerobic capacity.

There are multiple ways to conduct interval training, and I discuss a few of those methods here. To begin, most fighters execute interval training incorrectly. They go out as hard as they can each interval with their power output decreasing with each subsequent interval. This is called overreaching interval training, and it has a place within a well-designed program; however, the mistake many athletes make is that they conduct overreaching intervals every time they conduct intervals. The majority of your interval training should be executed so that the last interval is conducted at the same power output as the first interval but you can barely hold the output during the last interval. If you can barely hold the power output during the first interval, then your power output will continuously drop throughout the remaining interval. The first through last intervals should be performed at a level that is challenging but allows you to maintain the assigned power output for each interval.

Intervals can be performed in either long-time intervals or short-time intervals. You can execute short-time intervals of anywhere from 60 to 120 seconds each. If you pick 90 seconds for your intervals, each individual interval for that session will be conducted at 90 seconds. This type of interval really pushes your anaerobic abilities. You can also do longer interval sessions (5- to 10-minute intervals) that really work on pushing up your threshold.

Rest periods between intervals is another key concept to consider when executing interval training. You must make sure that energy systems and neuromuscular fatigue are addressed between bouts; however, there is no concrete evidence to state what the exact work-to-rest intervals should be at different interval time lengths. The typical recommendation is that the work-to-rest intervals for intervals that are 60 to 120 seconds should be about 1:3, and for intervals that are about 3 to 5 minutes, the work-to-rest intervals should be a 1:1 ratio. So, if you are conducting a 60-second interval (work), your recovery should be 180 seconds (rest). If you are carrying out 5-minute intervals (work), your recovery should be 5 minutes (rest). The rest interval can be performed either active (very easy walk/jog) or passive (no walking or jogging). Either will work, but I tend to recommend active recovery during long sessions. Keep in mind that active means you are walking/jogging very easily and slowly for recovery.

You can also conduct fartlek sessions, where the intervals are not timed specifically and instead you pick up the pace at random intervals and recover in between. Typically, I recommend that you feel well recovered but not necessarily completely recovered between intervals. This can be something fun you can do with your friends. Assign everyone a number, one through however many are running with you, and the intervals start in number order. Line up by number, and start the run. When the first runner decides to start the interval, they can quickly pick up speed without a word, and everyone else should attempt to keep up. During the recovery phase, the first runner goes to the back of the line, and then runner two should decide when to pick up the pace again. Keep repeating this process throughout the run.

Overreaching intervals can be used periodically to maximize stress on the physiological systems of your body. Unlike normal intervals, overreaching intervals will have continuously slower intervals as the training session progresses. Each interval is executed as fast as you can run, which will result in slower intervals as you fatigue with each subsequent interval. Overreaching intervals should be used sparingly, as they place high stress on the body.

FLEXIBILITY

Flexibility is your ability to move each joint through the complete range of motion for that particular joint. Flexibility is a major component of MMA and should be a founding principle of your training regimen. While flexibility is very important for the sport of MMA, it is often overlooked by many athletes, resulting in decreased performance and overuse injuries.

There are different methods used to increase flexibility. This book focuses on the two primary methods for improving flexibility and when to use them. The first method used to increase flexibility is called static stretching. When conducting a static stretch, slowly move into the proper position for that specific stretch and hold it for 10 to 30 seconds. When you move into the stretch, only go to the point of slight discomfort. Never go to the point of pain, as it is counterproductive, causing the muscle to tighten during the stretch.

The second form of stretching I am going to discuss is dynamic stretching. This form of stretching requires that you move through the full range of motion for that particular joint in a dynamic manner without holding a stretch. Dynamic stretching is used during warm-ups for competition to increase range of motion and optimize performance.

Both static and dynamic stretching have a place in your training and competition. There is much debate about whether static stretching is harmful prior to competition. Some research states that power and speed are reduced when static stretching is used prior to competition, as opposed to dynamic stretching; however, the current pool of research is not conclusive, and studies have not examined MMA, where flexibility is a primary component of competition. I would recommend static stretching, followed by dynamic stretching, going into your precompetition warm-up. Static stretching is key when it comes to increasing range of motion and should remain an integral part of your training program.

Static Stretches

As a mixed martial artist, you will place a lot of stress on your neck and surrounding muscles. When stretching the muscles of your neck, it is important to include rotation, flexion, extension, and lateral flexion.

- Begin by rotating to the left as far as the head will move and hold, and then repeat this process to the right.
- Take the neck into flexion by trying to touch your chin to your chest and hold the stretch. Next move the head into extension by rotating your chin toward the ceiling and hold.

- Take your head into lateral flexion to the right by taking your right ear toward your shoulder. Hold that position and then repeat this process to the left.
- When stretching the neck, it is important not to apply a large force or conduct these movements in a fast or bouncing movement.

Anterior Shoulder Stretch

This stretch is designed to stretch the anterior deltoid and pectoralis major. Abduct your arm until it is parallel to the floor, and place your hand on any object that will not move (e.g., a wall or door frame). Next rotate your upper body away from the arm that is being held in place, stretching the anterior muscles of the shoulder.

Posterior Shoulder Stretch

The posterior shoulder stretch focuses on the posterior deltoid and muscles of the back. Horizontally adduct your right arm across the chest, place your left hand on the elbow, and apply pressure to stretch.

Behind-the-Head Stretch

The behind-the-head stretch focuses on the triceps and latissimus dorsi. Raise your right arm above your head, and then flex at the elbow until your hand is behind your head. Reach up with your left hand, grab your elbow, and apply pressure to the left. Repeat this process with the left arm.

Abdominal Stretch

As the name indicates, this stretch focuses on the abdominal muscles. Lie prone (on your stomach), and place your hands palms down on the floor. Push upward with your arms, leaving your lower body flat on the floor.

Lower Body

Calf Stretch

The calf muscle (triceps surae) is made up of the gastrocnemius and soleus muscles. To stretch the calf muscle, stand on a raised surface with the fore part of the foot on the surface and the heel hanging off the surface. Allow the heel to go down by placing the foot in dorsiflexion. To concentrate on the gastrocnemius, keep the leg straight during this process. To focus more on the soleus, slightly flex at the knee, and repeat the process. Placing the knee into flexion places slack on the gastrocnemius and allows a greater focus on the soleus.

Hamstring Stretch

The basic hamstring stretch does much more than just stretch the hamstrings. This stretch is also great for the muscles of the lower back. If you can reach your toes and pull the foot into dorsiflexion, it will also stretch the calf. While this stretch can be executed standing, I advise conducting the stretch seated. Sit with your legs together and straight out in front of you. Bend forward at the waist, going as far forward and down as possible. Grab your toes and pull the foot into dorsiflexion. If you cannot reach your toes, grab as far down the leg as you can. Keep your legs straight, and do not allow a lot of bend at the knee.

Modified Hurdle Stretch

The modified hurdle stretch primarily focuses on the hamstrings and muscles of the lower back (see figure 3.1). Sit on your bottom with your left leg straight

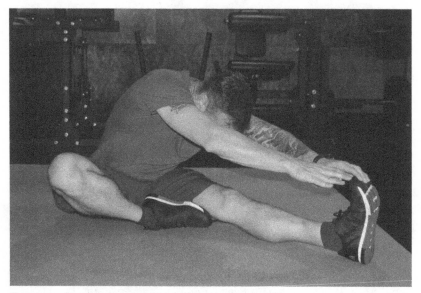

Figure 3.1. Modified Hurdle Stretch

out in front of you and your right leg flexed at the knee with the bottom of your foot in contact with your left leg. Bend forward and attempt to place both hands on your left foot. Repeat this stretch with the right side.

Straddle Stretch

The saddle stretch primarily focuses on the hamstrings, adductor muscles, and muscles of the lower back. Sit on your bottom with your legs spread wide (horizontal split). Lean your body over your left leg, attempting to touch your foot with your right hand, and then repeat the movement on your right leg. Once you have completed those movements, bend toward the floor in the middle.

Quadriceps Stretch

The quadriceps stretch is typically executed incorrectly by trying to push the heel into the gluteus maximus while in flexion. Instead, reach behind the body and grab the right leg with the left hand, place the knee into flexion, and pull rearward. Repeat this process with the other leg. If you have trouble balancing on one leg during this process, move to a wall and place your free hand on the wall for balance.

Adductor Stretch

The adductor stretch (butterfly stretch) focuses on the adductor muscles. Sit on the floor and place the knees into flexion with the soles of the feet touching. Grab your feet and place your elbows on your legs. Push down on your legs with your elbows and bend forward at the waist.

Hip Stretch

The hip stretch focuses on the gluteus maximus and hamstrings. Lie supine (on your back) with both legs straight out. Bring your right leg up by flexing at the hip. As you bring the leg up, allow the knee to go into flexion. Place your hands behind the knee and pull. Repeat this process with the left leg.

Supine Twist

The supine stretch focuses on the muscles around the spine and the external oblique and gluteus muscles (see figure 3.2). Lay on your left side, keeping your left leg straight and bending your right knee. Your left arm should be perpendicular to your body and laying on the ground with your right arm on top of the left. Keeping your right leg in place, rotate your upper body toward the right, placing your shoulders flat on the ground. Your right arm should now be on the ground and perpendicular to your body. Repeat this process on your right side.

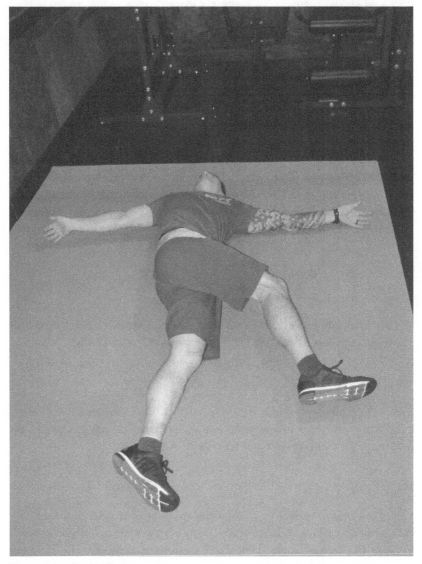

Figure 3.2. Supine Twist

Side Split

The side split focuses primarily on the adductor muscles. Not everyone's anthropometrics are optimal for easily achieving a full split. Even if you are not going all the way to the floor with the side splits, you are still gaining flexibility. Side splits are designed to allow you to kick higher (primarily the side kick and the round kick). To conduct side splits, use your hands on the ground to control your descent into the split. As your legs slide apart, make sure you only go to mild discomfort and that you are feeling no pain in the hips or knees.

Front Split

The front split focuses on the hamstrings and gluteus maximus in the front leg, and the rectus femoris, psoas major, tensor fascia latae, and sartorius. The front split differs from the side split in that one leg will go forward as the other leg goes back. Front splits are designed to increase flexibility during a push kick (teep) and a front kick. To conduct a front split, use your hands to support your weight as your left leg moves outward in front of your body and your back right leg moves backward behind your body. Repeat on the opposite side. Make sure to move slowly into the stretch, and do not force it.

Dynamic Stretches

Wrist Rotations

Wrist rotations are performed by rotating both wrists counterclockwise for about 15 seconds and then reversing to clockwise for another 15 seconds.

Cross-Body Arm Swings

To conduct cross-body arm swings horizontally, abduct your arms and then adduct them across your chest with one arm slightly above the other as they cross. Alternate which arm is above and below with each swing.

Elbow Circles

For elbow circles, abduct your arms slightly from your sides and focus the circles from the elbow. You will not actually have rotation at the elbow, it will be more like circumduction with slight shoulder movement. Start by going counterclockwise for 15 seconds and then clockwise for another 15 seconds.

Arm Circles

For arm circles, rotate your arms from the shoulders in a 360-degree circle (circumduction). Conduct arm rotations to the front for 15 seconds, and then rotate them to the back for 15 seconds.

Trunk Rotation

To execute trunk rotation, place your feet a little wider than shoulder-width apart and abduct your arms until they are approximately parallel to the floor, and then rotate as far as you can go to the left and then back to the right as far as you can go.

Butt Kicks

Butt kicks can be conducted in place, walking, or jogging. As your foot comes off the ground, drive the heel to your butt with each step. Alternate legs as you execute the dynamic stretch. When you first start this movement, your heel may not reach your butt. This is okay, just get your heel as high as you can.

High Knees

High knees can be conducted in place, walking, or jogging. When the foot leaves the ground, bring your knee as high as possible toward your chest. Alternate legs as you execute the dynamic stretch.

High Knee Hip Circles

Conduct this movement in place. Bring your knee up high toward your chest, and then rotate away from your body and back to the ground, landing in your starting position. Alternate legs as you execute this movement. After 15 seconds, reverse this movement (rotate from the outside in).

Leg Swings

You can execute leg swings with or without support. If you need support for balance, place your hand on a wall or nonmoveable object. Without bending your knee, kick your leg forward as high as possible, and then allow it to swing down and behind you as far as possible. After 15 seconds switch to the other leg, and conduct leg swings for another 15 seconds.

Lateral Leg Swings

Lateral leg swings are executed similar to leg swings, but instead of front to back, you swing your leg from side to side (abduct and adduct). Kick your leg to the side, and then allow it to come down and cross in front of your stationary leg. After 15 seconds, switch to the other leg, and conduct leg swings for another 15 seconds.

Supine Leg Circle

To conduct supine leg circles, lay on your back and bend at the hips until your thighs are perpendicular to the floor, and then move your feet in a circle. Move your left foot clockwise and your right foot counterclockwise. After 15 seconds, reverse each foot for another 15 seconds.

RESISTANCE TRAINING FOR MUSCULAR ENDURANCE, MUSCULAR STRENGTH, AND MUSCULAR POWER

Muscular Endurance

Muscular endurance is the body's ability to contract repeatedly or continuously. Muscular endurance is often tested using such activities as push-ups, pull-ups, and sit-ups. The goal of muscular endurance is to increase the number of repetitions that you do with each exercise. During training and competition, you will be required to conduct multiple contractions using the same muscles; therefore, increasing muscular endurance will improve your MMA performance. Here I describe a few of the most common muscular endurance exercises that you can implement into your program. Also, keep in mind that you can conduct muscular endurance exercises with low weight and high reps (15–25) using the exercises described in the "Resistance Training" section.

Muscular Strength

Muscular strength is defined as the maximal amount of force a muscle can produce at one time. To increase muscular strength, low reps (4–8) and heavy weights are used during resistance training. It is important to be as strong as possible within your weight class. There is nothing more frustrating than to be overpowered by an opponent with a lower level of technique. If your and your opponent's techniques are equivalent, being stronger gives you an edge.

Muscular strength is frequently measured by conducting a one-repetition maximum (1RM) test. A 1RM test is most commonly conducted for the bench press, squat, and dead lift. It is designed to monitor your progression throughout your training program. At the completion of the strength training phase of your program, you should see an increase in your 1RM in relation to your 1RM at the beginning of the strength training phase.

These tests should only be conducted with experienced lifters who have a good strength base and a strong grasp of proper lifting technique. Use of improper technique during a 1RM can result in serious injury. Moreover, conducting a 1RM without a good base will result in serious delayed onset of muscle soreness (DOMS), which could negatively impact the rest of the scheduled training for the week.

To conduct a 1RM, you should be well rested and injury free. Make sure that you have sufficient spotters. You may need multiple spotters, depending on the weight. Use a warm-up weight that allows you to easily conduct 10 to 12 repetitions. Rest for about 2 to 5 minutes. After completing the first warm-up set and rest period, increase the resistance to a weight that is about 75 to 85 percent of your previous 1RM. If you do not have a previous 1RM, use a weight that allows you to conduct 8 repetitions. Then rest for 2 to 5 minutes. Now you are ready to attempt your 1RM. If you have a previous 1RM, that is where you will start. If you do not have a previous 1RM, you will increase by about 20 percent of your 8-repetition set you just completed. You want to slowly increase weight for each attempt until you cannot complete the lift. You should rest 5 minutes between each attempt to allow for recovery. If you are doing multiple lifts (bench, dead lift, squat, etc.) conduct them in the same order each time you conduct a 1RM session.

Muscular Power

Muscular power is how quickly you can move a given resistance. Power is derived from the force required to move a resistance multiplied by the distance the resistance traveled and then divided by the time required to complete the move. Simplified: Muscular power = muscular force × velocity of movement. Muscular strength accounts for the force portion of the formula and is an important component; however, the second part of the formula, how quickly the movement occurs, is key. If one fighter can move the same weight in half the time of another fighter, that fighter produced twice the power (assuming both fighters moved the weight the exact same distance). Power is a key component for just about any move in MMA, as the fighter wants to generate force as quickly as possible. While strength is a key component of power, training power is where you will see a large improvement in your striking power.

Keep in mind that correct striking techniques are key to power, and you must have this key factor correct before improving muscular power through training. For power strikes, force is generated from the ground up, and your power increases as you learn to use this concept when throwing strikes. This is why you pivot from the ground with any power strike you throw. Once you have your technique down, you will see improvements in power from training to improve muscular power. Training muscular power, in and of itself, will not greatly improve your striking power if your technique is poor.

To develop power, you need to work on muscle activation speed. Naturally, speed will increase for a specific movement (punching, kicking, elbows, etc.) as you develop the correct neuromuscular recruitment patterns from repetitive practice of that particular movement; however, in this section we are focusing on increasing speed, and therefore power, through strength and conditioning methods. One of the easiest methods to implement for improved power is the use of plyometrics. Plyometric movements consist of an eccentric load followed by a powerful concentric contraction and are very dynamic. Box jumps are an example of plyometrics. More complicated movements, for instance, a power clean or snatch, are great for power development but are beyond the scope of this book, as you would need a coach to critique your form to prevent injury. Plyometrics are easy to learn, easy to implement, and produce great results.

Resistance Training

It is important that you learn the proper technique for every lift and movement you plan on using in your resistance program. The use of improper technique is one of the most common causes of injury in the weight room. You want to lift in a controlled manner that precisely follows the correct technique. While each lift requires specific techniques, there are general guidelines that go with every lift. They are as follows:

- Maintain proper technique throughout the movements. Don't try to use momentum to get through a lift where the resistance is too heavy. If the resistance is heavy enough to require you to alter proper form, you should decrease the weight to maintain form.
- Movements should be conducted in a controlled manner and at a constant speed. The speed should not be explosive and fast (unless you are conducting specific plyometric training), nor should it be super slow.

- Correctly grip the bar at all times to prevent the bar from rolling out of your hands.
- Do not attempt to lift weights that are too heavy for your current fitness level. This is a common source of injury. Remember to let your ego go. It does not matter how much you are lifting. You are not training to be a powerlifter. You are training to be the best fighter you can become.
- Work large muscle groups before working small muscle groups. If you work the small muscle groups first, they will become too fatigued to allow you to adequately work the large muscle groups. For example, if you work the triceps brachii first and then work the pectoralis major, the triceps will be too fatigued and give out prior to the pectoralis major fatiguing. Instead, work the pectoralis major first and then the triceps.
- Never hold your breath. Inhale during the eccentric load, and exhale during the concentric load. Holding your breath during a lift will result in a larger spike in blood pressure than normal (blood pressure always spikes during lifting), which will cause a large decrease in blood pressure when the lift stops, resulting in dizziness.
- For safety, always use a spotter with free weights.
- Use collars on barbells to keep the weight from shifting on the bar. It only takes a slight shift in the bar to cause a weight to slide, resulting in a catastrophic event as the plates start sliding off the bar.

One of your first steps is to determine frequency by setting the length of the program and how many days per week you will use resistance training. The length of each phase of your resistance training will be dependent on the goal of that phase. For example, you will have a strength-building phase that will last four to eight weeks, followed by a power-building phase that will last four to eight weeks. This concept is discussed in detail in the following chapter. Resistance training should be conducted two to three days per week depending on your training goals and which training phase you are in.

The next step is to determine your sets and repetitions. Sets are the number of times you perform the exercise, and repetition is the number of times you lift or perform the movement per set. You will want to keep your sets between two and three for most all of your exercises. You may want to go up to four or five for muscular endurance or plyometrics. The repetition of the exercises will be determined by the training phase you are in. If your goal is strength development, your resistance will be high and your reps low (3–6 repetitions). If your goal is power development, you will lower the weight and increase the repetitions (8–12 repetitions). Keep in mind that during the power development phase, you will be conducting plyometrics at high repetitions. If the focus is on muscular endurance, the repetitions will be greater than 12.

Determine weight based on desired repetitions. For example, if you are conducting two sets with goal repetitions of 8 to 12, you would set the weight so that volitional exhaustion occurs between 8 and 12 reps for both sets. If you are able to conduct more than 12 repetitions, then increase the weight. If you cannot conduct at least 8 repetitions, then decrease the weight. When choosing a weighted ball for plyometrics, make sure that you start off with a lighter ball and then move your way up so that you can achieve the desired repetitions.

The next step is to choose the resistance exercises. The following are examples of exercises that you can implement in your resistance training program. If you are serious about your performance, consider hiring a strength and conditioning coach with a background in MMA performance.

Work your entire body, including the upper body, lower body, and core; avoid focusing on one area and ignoring others. The lifts and exercises listed here supply a sufficient program to cover all the major muscle groups that are important to a mixed martial artist. You will not have to use all the resistance exercises listed during a single training session. Instead, choose the exercises that work best to achieve your desired outcome. You can replace these exercises with others that work the same muscles or focus more on a specific area by adding different exercises into your program. If you are not familiar with the muscles involved in each specific exercise, I strongly recommend purchasing a book that shows the specific muscles used in each movement.

When lifting, start with large muscle groups and then follow up with small muscles. For example, work bench press prior to working triceps. If you fatigue the triceps by conducting triceps extensions prior to doing bench, you will not be able to adequately work the pectoralis major due to triceps fatigue.

Resistance Exercises

Bench Press

The pectoralis major, anterior deltoid, and triceps brachii are the primary muscles used in the bench press (see figure 3.3). Other muscles used during the bench press are the anterior deltoids, serratus anterior, and coracobrachialis. To execute the bench press, lie flat on your back with both feet planted on the floor. Place your hands on the bar about shoulder-width apart with the palms facing away and fingers and thumbs wrapped around the bar. Begin by lowering the weight until it is about one inch from your chest. Do not bounce the weight

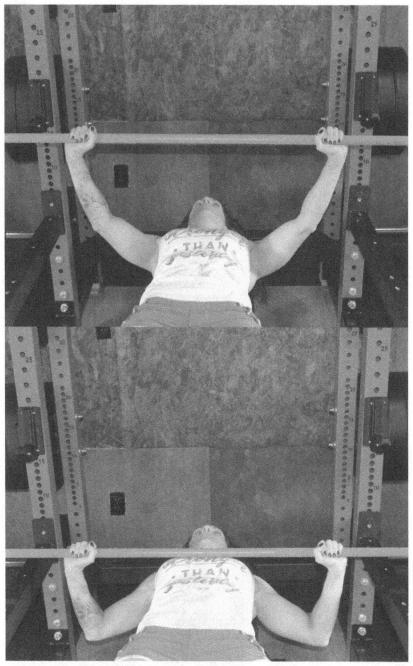

Figure 3.3.   Bench Press

off your chest. From the lowered position, push the weight back up to the start position.

Lat Pulldowns

The lat pulldown is designed to work the latissimus dorsi, teres major, and biceps brachii (see figure 3.4). Adjust the lat pulldown machine per the manufacturer's instructions. Grab the bar just wider than shoulder width so that your

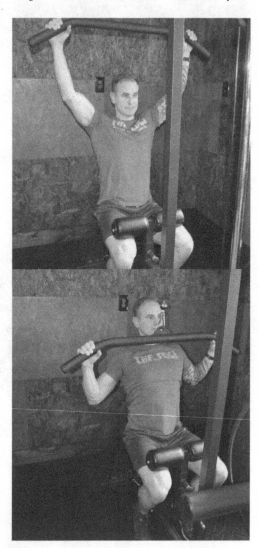

Figure 3.4.   Lat Pulldowns

palms are facing away from you. Pull the bar down in front of your head and then return to the start position.

Seated Rows

The latissimus dorsi, trapezius, rhomboid (major and minor), teres major, posterior deltoids, and biceps brachii are worked during the seated row (see figure 3.5). Adjust the machine per the manufacturer's instructions. Begin by bringing

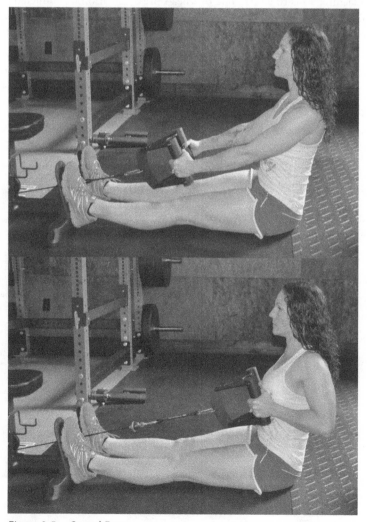

Figure 3.5.   Seated Rows

the bar/handles to your chest and then returning to the start position. Maintain proper back posture throughout the movement.

Overhead Press

The overhead press can be conducted either seated or standing (see figure 3.6). The deltoid, pectoralis major (clavicular head only), and triceps are the primary muscles used during this exercise. When performed on a machine, follow the manufacturer's instructions. The overhead press can also be conducted using dumbbells. Grab the dumbbells in an overhand grip, and place the dumbbells a little higher than shoulder level with the back of the hand facing you. This is the start position. Press up over the head and then return to the start position. The overhead press can be conducted with a barbell, but I recommend that beginners stick with dumbbells. Dumbbells allow for more natural joint movement throughout the lift.

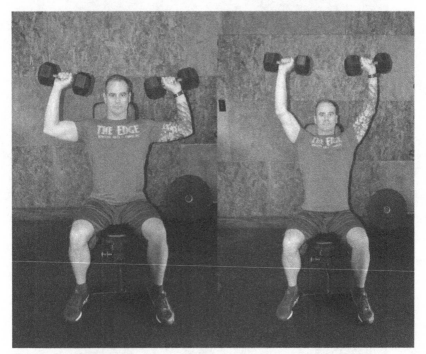

Figure 3.6.   Overhead Press

Squats

The primary muscles used during the squat are the quadriceps, hamstrings, and gluteus maximus (see figure 3.7). The first step in conducting the squat is to adjust the squat rack height so that you can easily take the bar off and put it back when the set is complete. When conducting the squat, center the bar across the back and shoulders, and grab the bar with both hands. Choose a hand position that provides both comfort and control of the bar. Lift the bar off the rack and back up into position, making sure to stay over the safety bars. Place your feet shoulder-width apart. During the lowering phase, do not allow your knees to move forward beyond your feet. Lower into the squatted position until your thighs are parallel to the floor. Push up with the legs, returning to the standing position. When pushing up, drive through your heels, keeping the weight centered. When you reach the top of the lift, do not lock your knees. To maintain proper posture, make sure you do not look down with your head, as it will shift your center of gravity forward. Keep your head looking forward or slightly up and drive with your heels.

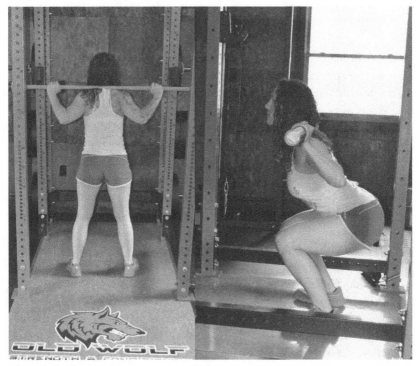

Figure 3.7.   Squats

Leg Extensions

Leg extensions focus on the muscles of the quadriceps (rectus femoris, vastus intermedius, vastus lateralis, and vastus medialis). Before beginning leg extensions, ensure that the machine you are working on is set up specifically for you. Do not lock your knees at the top of the knee extension.

Leg Curls

Leg curls are designed to strengthen the hamstrings (semitenndinosus, semimembanosis, and biceps femoris). Because the gastrocnemius crosses the knee, it will be worked along with the hamstring muscles. Adjust the leg curl machine in accordance with the manufacturer's instructions. Leg curls (as well as leg extensions) typically are not recommended for sports performance because they are isolation exercises; however, anterior cruciate ligament (ACL) injuries are quite common in MMA. One of the recommended methods for preventing ACL injuries is to ensure that you have as little strength discrepancies as possible between the quadriceps and the hamstring muscles.

Dead Lifts

Dead lifts primarily focus on the gluteus maximus, hamstring muscles, quadriceps, erector spinae, rhomboids, and trapezius (see figure 3.8). When conducting the dead lift, I recommend using a hex bar (trap bar) as opposed to a straight bar. When using a straight bar, it is important to keep the bar as close to the shins as possible. This often leads to beat up and gouged shins. The hex bar also puts your trunk in a more upright position and slightly reduces the risk of lower back injury. For those with lower back issues, most hex bars will have a higher handle that allows you to start from a higher position. Lastly, you are not competing in a powerlifting competition; therefore, a straight-bar dead lift is not required. With the exception of slightly different knee angles and trunk angle, all other angles are the same, and the work between a straight-bar dead lift and a hex-bar dead lift is the same (even though you can lift more with a hex bar). The center of gravity alters with a hex bar and allows for a more comfortable lift.

To conduct a hex-bar dead lift, step into the hex bar with your feet about shoulder-width apart. Grab the bar and align it so that the center of the bar and the center of the hands are at the midpoint of the ankle. When you grab the bar, do not bend at the waist and instead squat down. Drive the bar up from the feet, and do not lift with the back. Thrust your hips forward as you come up (do not overexaggerate). During the eccentric phase (lowering back to the ground),

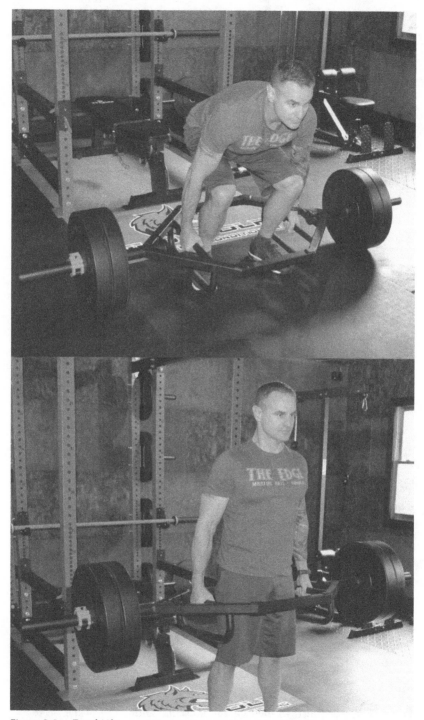

Figure 3.8. Dead Lifts

make sure that the weights hit the floor evenly. If the weights touch the floor unevenly, you need to either slow down or drop weight so that you can move smoothly through the motion, with both sides of the weight touching the floor at the same time.

Hip Thrusters

Hip thrusters focus primarily on the hamstrings and gluteus maximus (see figure 3.9). This exercise mimics a bridge and upa (you have to bridge high prior to turning into the upa). This exercise can be done with and without weights. If you are just beginning, start without weights. Begin by sitting on the ground and placing your upper back on the bench. Once you have established this position, roll the barbell into place across your waist. If you have bony hips, you may want a towel or pad to prevent the bar from digging in. Bend your knees to about 90 degrees with your feet about shoulder-width apart. Place your hands on the bar to stabilize and lift your bottom off the ground. Once in this position, adjust your feet so that your shins are perpendicular to the floor. Tuck your chin to your chest, and then lower the weight at the hips and bridge back up into position. Do not use heavy weights or jerking motions during this exercise, as both could result in back injuries. If you are conducting hip thrusters without weights you can do single-leg thrusts to increase resistance.

Muscular Endurance Exercises

Pull-ups

The pull-up is designed to improve the muscular endurance of the latissimus dorsi, teres major, and biceps brachii (see figure 3.10). The rhomboids are also worked when the shoulder blades are pulled together at the top of the pull-up. Grasp the pull-up bar a little wider than shoulder width with the hands facing away from you. In the start position, you will be hanging with your arms straight and no weight on the ground. Pull your body weight toward the bar until the chin clears the bar, and then return to the start position. Do not use a swinging motion during this movement. If you want to improve grip strength, you can do dial rod pull-ups.

Push-ups

Push-ups are designed to increase the muscular endurance of the pectoralis major, anterior deltoid, and triceps brachii (see figure 3.11). Lie facedown on

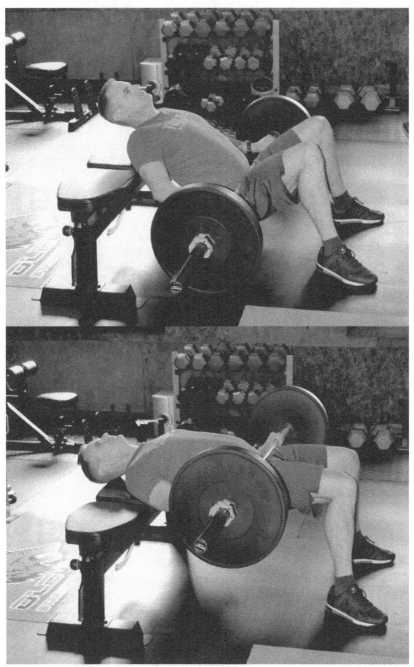

Figure 3.9. Hip Thrusters

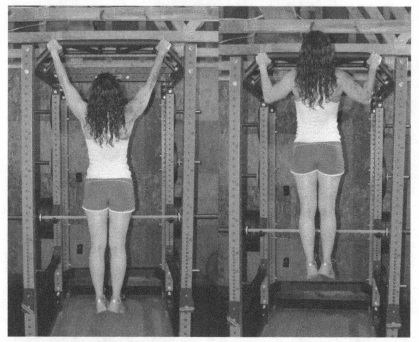

Figure 3.10.   Pull-ups

the floor, placing the hands just wider than the shoulders. From this position, push up until the arms are straight. This is the start position. From the start position, lower your body until the elbows are at approximately a 90-angle and return to the start position. The weight should be borne by the hands and the toes throughout the movement, and the body should stay straight as well. If you are just beginning, you can perform a modified push-up by changing the contact point from the toes to the knees.

Dips

Dips are designed to work primarily the pectoralis major, triceps, and anterior deltoid (see figure 3.12). This movement is typically conducted on dip bars. Start with your arms at your side and extended at the elbow. Lower your body until your chest is even with the dip bars and push back up. You can alter the percentage activation of the pectoralis and triceps by leaning your body. The more vertical you are, the more the triceps will be activated, and the more you lean forward, the more the pectoralis major will be activated.

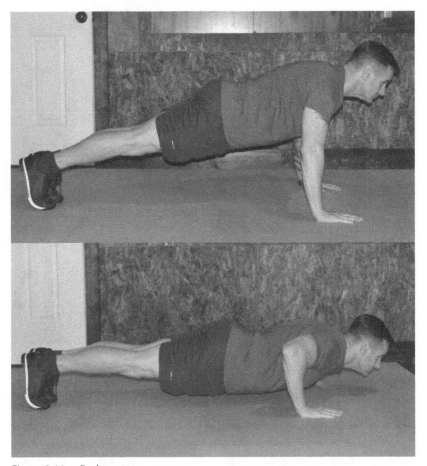

Figure 3.11.   Push-ups

Horizontal Rows

The horizontal row primarily focuses on the latissimus dorsi, rhomboids, trapezius, posterior deltoid, and biceps brachii (see figure 3.13). To conduct this exercise, you will need a horizontal bar (a power rack and barbell will work) and a bench. From underneath grab the bar with your hands a little wider than shoulder-width apart, and place your feet on the bench. Keeping your body in a straight line, pull up on the bar until your chest touches and then lower back down until your arms are straight.

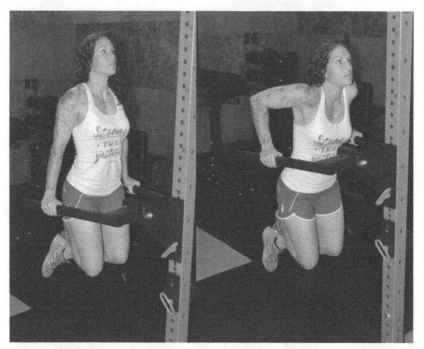

Figure 3.12.   Dips

Lunges

The primary muscles involved in lunges are the quadriceps, hamstrings, and gluteus maximus (see figure 3.14). Lunges can be conducted weighted or without weight. Beginners should start by conducting lunges with no weights and move to weighted lunges only when are ready.

Start by placing your feet about shoulder-width apart. Step forward with your right leg, and lower your body until the thigh of the right leg is parallel to the floor and the knee of the left leg is almost touching the floor. Return to the standing position, and repeat this process by stepping forward with the left leg. Lunges can also be conducted in a walking manner by leaving the lead foot planted and bringing the rear leg forward into a lunge.

Army Crawl

When conducting the army low crawl, lie prone with your weight on your forearms and lower body with your left knee bent and toward your left elbow

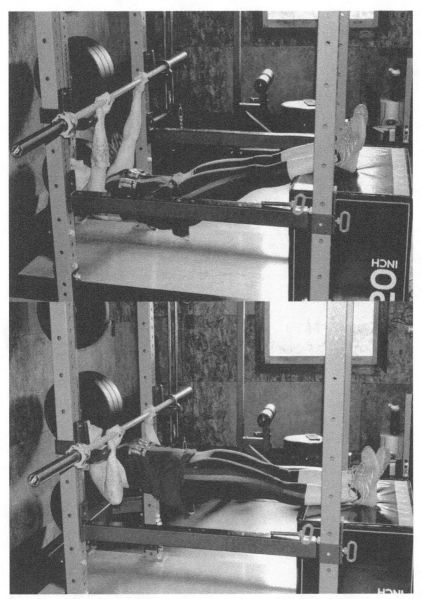

Figure 3.13.　Horizontal Rows

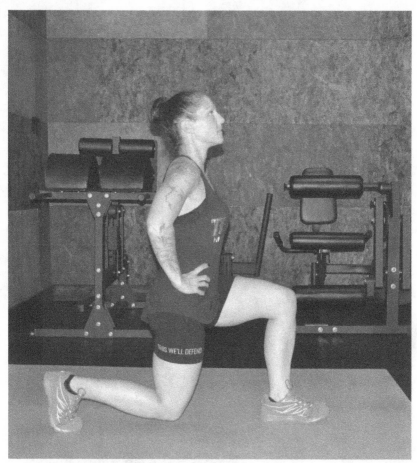

Figure 3.14.   Lunges

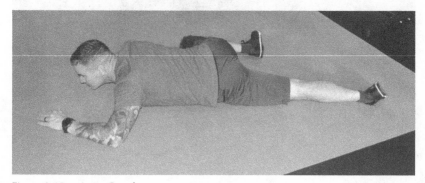

Figure 3.15.   Army Crawl

(see figure 3.15). Move your right arm forward, and push off with your left leg and bring your right leg up and your left arm up as your body moves forward. Repeat this process on the opposite side.

Alligator Crawl

To perform the alligator crawl, begin in a push-up position (see figure 3.16). Bring your left leg toward and past your left elbow (on the outside of the arm) as you reach forward with your right arm while lowering your body almost to the floor. From this position you will push up as you lift your left hand and right foot. Move your left hand forward and your right knee toward and past your right elbow, and lower to the ground as your left hand and right foot make contact. Repeat this process for the other side.

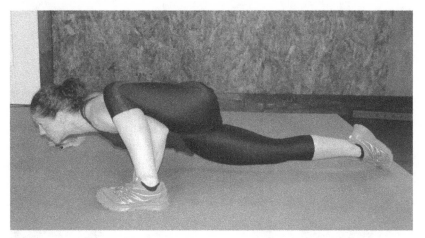

Figure 3.16.   Alligator Crawl

Bear Crawl

To execute the bear crawl, position yourself with your hands, knees, and feet on the ground, and your back straight and flat (see figure 3.17). Lift your knees off the ground to the point where your shins are about parallel to the floor, with your back remaining straight. Maintain a straight back, and do not put your butt high in the air. Walk forward by moving your left hand and right foot forward at the same time. You do not want to take large steps forward like with the alligator crawl. Instead, keep your legs in line with the arms. Repeat this process with the opposite leg and arm.

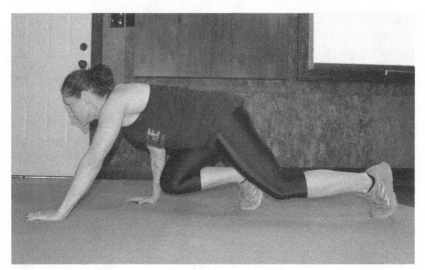

Figure 3.17.   Bear Crawl

Burpees

Burpees are not only a good exercise, but also required in some obstacle course races (see figure 3.18). While I am listing the burpee as a muscular endurance exercise, the move can also be considered a plyometric exercise, due to the explosive nature. There are different variations to the burpee, but I am going to cover the basic burpee.

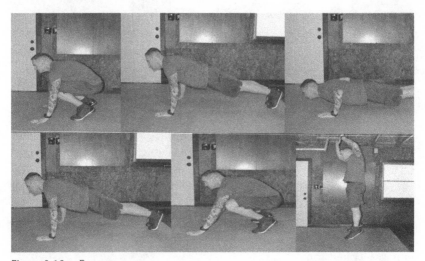

Figure 3.18.   Burpees

Begin with your legs slightly shoulder-width apart. Squat down, place your hands shoulder-width apart on the ground, and shoot your legs out to a push-up position. Next execute a push-up, bring your legs back under you to the squat position, and jump high into the air. Repeat.

Core Exercises

It is important that the core muscles work to stabilize the spine and pelvis during many movements in MMA. There is a common misconception that the core muscles are primarily just the abdominal muscles and erector spinae muscles; however, the core is correctly defined as the multitude of muscles (approximately 29) designed to stabilize the pelvis and spine. The core muscles are worked during all of the previously described lifting movements to stabilize the spine and pelvis throughout the lift. I am, however, going to describe common exercises that focus on the abdominals and erector spinae. Those truly interested in developing a workout to develop core muscular endurance can expand this portion of their workout by adding more exercises.

Crunches

Crunches are designed to focus on the rectus abdominis and the oblique abdominals. Lie with your back on the floor, and place your legs in the air, bending at the hips and knees. You can also conduct the crunch by placing your heels on a bench. Place your arms across your chest, and curl your body off the floor until the upper back is clear of the floor. Repeat for as many reps as possible. After completing a normal set of normal crunches, you can add in a set of twisting crunches. From the same start position, curl up, twisting your right shoulder to your left knee, and return to the start position. On the next rep, curl up, twisting the left shoulder to the right knee, and then return to the start position. Repeat this sequence until exhaustion.

Leg Raises

The leg raise is designed to work the abdominal muscles and hip flexor muscles. Lie on your back with your head off the floor, arms at your side, and feet just off the floor. Lift your legs just past 90 degrees of hip flexion and return to the start position. Keep your legs straight throughout this process.

Hanging Leg Raises

Hanging leg raises are designed to work the abdominal muscles and the hip flexor muscles (see figure 3.19). Hang from a bar or rings with your arms straight, and curl up with your abdominal muscles as you bring your knees to your chest. You can twist to your left and right as you come up to focus more on the obliques.

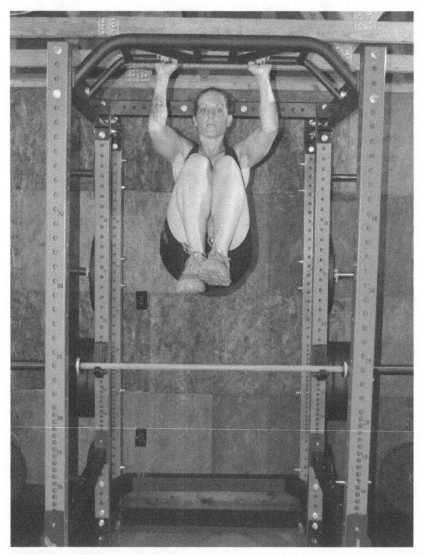

Figure 3.19.   Hanging Leg Raises

Back Extensions

Back extensions work the erector spinae muscles (see figure 3.20). Lie face-down on the floor with your toes pointed, and place your hands behind your head or straight out in front of you. Begin by lifting your upper body off of the floor, and return to the start position. You can either keep your lower body in contact with the floor or lift it from the floor in unison with the upper body to add glutes and hamstring muscles.

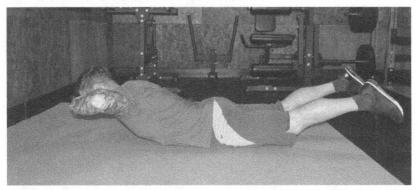

Figure 3.20.   Back Extensions

Roman Chair Back Extensions

The roman chair back extension works the erector spinae muscles, glutes, and hamstring muscles (see figure 3.21). Adjust the roman chair so that the ankles are under the pad and the thighs are on the support pads. Place your hands on or by your ears, and bend forward at the waist and then extend your back upward.

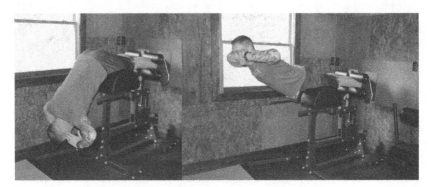

Figure 3.21.   Roman Chair Back Extensions

Plyometrics

Plyometrics are an important tool that will allow you to increase power upon completion of your strength phase. A plyometric exercise uses the stretch-shortening cycle to produce a more powerful movement. The stretch-shortening cycle involves an eccentric load that is stretched and then followed up by a powerful concentric contraction. An example of a plyometric movement is when you squat down prior to a jump. When you squat down you are stretching the eccentrically loaded muscles, and the concentric contraction occurs when you jump up from the squat. One of the things that makes a cross so powerful after a jab is that the jab turns the body to the right (if you are fighting orthodox). This puts the muscles into the eccentric load that allows you to come back from the right with a cross that is more powerful. Adding plyometrics to your workout routine will allow you to better use the stretch-shortening cycle to strike and move with greater power.

When adding in plyometrics, it is important to start slowly due to the heavy eccentric loads. As in all other workouts, it is important to make sure you are using the correct techniques. Later in this chapter I will discuss a few of the basic lower and upper body techniques that you can use in your training. There are many more valid plyometric exercises that can be used as well.

Box Jumps

When conducting box jumps, it is important to choose a height that you can easily accomplish (see figure 3.22). While increasing height is how you will increase intensity, you want to make sure you can complete the desired number of repetitions prior to increasing height. Before beginning box jumps, I recommend conducting plyometric jumps from a flat surface. This will allow you to become accustomed to plyometrics before adding in the height of the box. Any jumps that you can do on the box you can also do without a box. If you choose to purchase a plyometric jump box, I suggest buying a foam box, as they are more forgiving on your shins in relation to metal or wood boxes.

Begin by standing close enough to the box so that you can easily make the jump, and place your feet about shoulder-width apart. Make sure that you have enough space so that you do not hit the box on the way up. Squat down, moving your arms behind you (countermovement), and then jump up, landing with both feet in the center of the box. Jump down and repeat. If you want to increase the intensity of the workout, you can add a depth jump when you step off the box. To add the depth jump, step off the box, land on both feet, squat down,

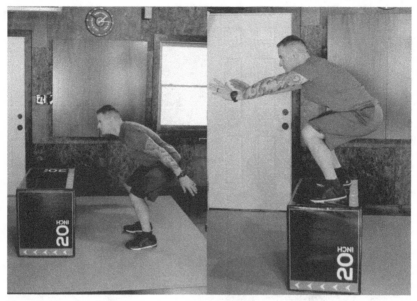

Figure 3.22. Box Jumps

and jump again. Each of these movements should be completed in a controlled and fluid motion.

Lateral Box Jumps

Begin by standing next to the box so that your left side is facing the box (see figure 3.23). Make sure that you are close enough to the box to easily make the jump but far enough away that you do not hit the box on the way up. Squat down, moving your arms behind you (countermovement), and jump laterally, landing on the box. Step down on the opposite side and repeat the process going the other way.

Chest Passes

When conducting upper body plyometrics, the use of a plyometric ball provides an optimal workout. Plyometric balls, also referred to as slam balls, wall balls, and medicine balls, come in different weights and styles. Some balls are made to bounce, while others are made to minimize bounce. Each type works. You will need to find which kind you prefer. Plyometric balls come in different weights. Choose a weight that allows you to complete the desired number of repetitions, while maintaining correct technique.

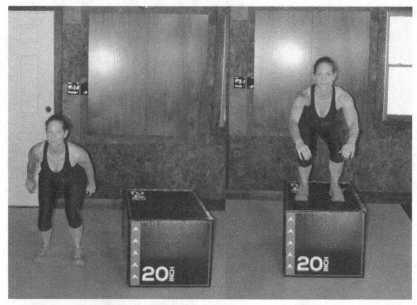

Figure 3.23.   Lateral Box Jumps

The chest pass can be performed individually or with a partner. If you are conducting the chest pass individually, you will need to find a wall that will not be damaged when the ball makes contact. If working with a partner, they will catch the ball and chest pass it back to you. If the weight of the ball makes it difficult for your partner to safely catch it, take turns on a wall.

Begin by placing your feet about shoulder-width apart. Bring the ball to your chest, creating the eccentric load, and push the ball away in a quick concentric contraction (see figure 3.24). If you are working with a partner, you will use the eccentric load from the catch to immediately pass the ball back to your partner.

Side Throws

Begin by standing in your fighting stance (orthodox) facing the wall. Hold the ball in both hands, and twist to the right, creating the eccentric load (see figure 3.25). Follow up with a strong concentric contraction, and release the ball as you twist to the left. Repeat this process for the opposite side of the body (southpaw).

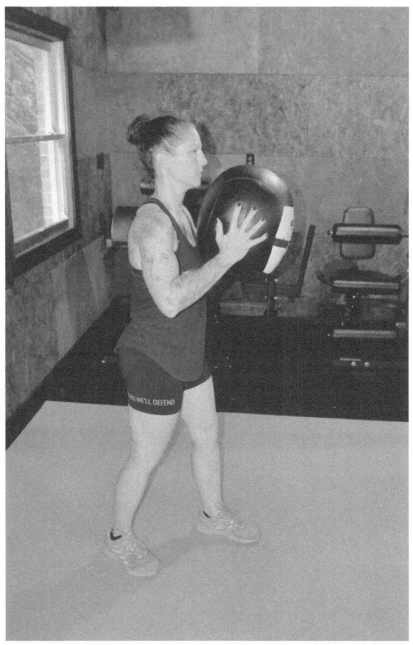

Figure 3.24.   Chest Passes

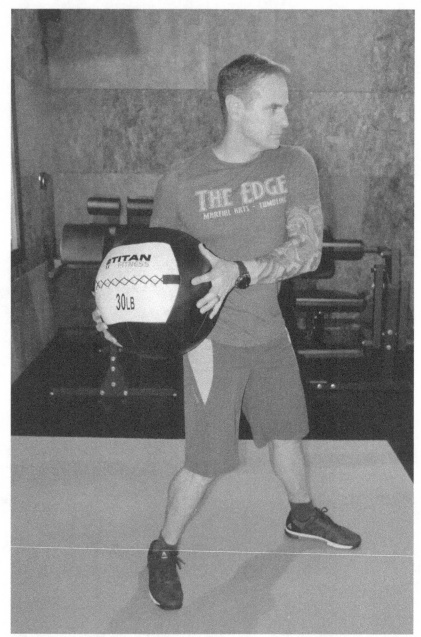

Figure 3.25.   Side Throws

Overhead Slams

Begin by placing your feet about shoulder-width apart. Bring the ball above your head, creating the eccentric load (see figure 3.26). Next, contract concentrically to slam the ball into the floor. You may want to choose a nonbouncing

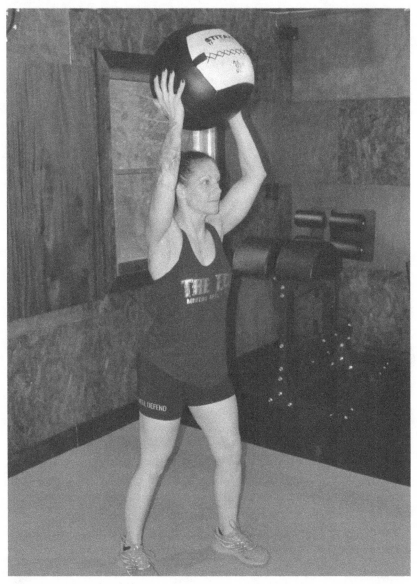

Figure 3.26.　Overhead Slams

plyometric ball for this exercise. A plyometric ball that bounces can easily bounce up and hit you in the face. On the other hand, if you are careful, you can use a bouncing plyometric ball and catch it on the way back up, as opposed to picking up a nonbouncing ball off the floor for every repetition.

Squat Throws

Begin by placing your feet a little wider than shoulder-width apart. Squat down with the ball in both hands and between your legs, creating the eccentric load (see figure 3.27). Drive through your heels and upward with your legs as you bring the ball up with your arms until your arms are above your head. Release the ball so that it is over your head and flying behind you after release.

Stair Workouts

Stair workouts can be done to increase power, aerobic capacity, or anaerobic capacity, or a combination of the three. If you choose to add a stair workout into your training program, you must keep these factors in mind. Running stairs at a slow pace you can handle is more of an aerobic workout; however, for most individuals, if you are running stairs, it will be at a higher intensity and therefore will be an anaerobic workout. Keep in mind that plyometrics are still involved but not optimized during an anaerobic workout.

To make it a plyometric workout, you will need to decrease the speed and focus on the plyometric aspects. Instead of running, you could double leg hop, single leg hop, and so on, at a slow pace, focusing on the plyometric aspect. You could even focus on sport-specific aspect by adding in kicks as you climb. For example, you could throw a teep (push kick), landing it on a step in front of you, and then push off into a single leg jump from the kicking leg, after it lands on the step. You can either alternate legs as you progress up the steps or do one side the first time up and switch to the opposite side the second time up.

When conducting stair workouts there are a few things to keep in mind. The first is that stairs are constructed of hard material and are very unforgiving on the body. Always proceed carefully. Make sure that your shoes are tied securely prior to beginning your session, and check them periodically throughout. Keep your focus on your technique throughout, and if you become too fatigued to maintain proper technique, it's time to quit for the day. Most accidents occur because the athlete becomes too fatigued to conduct the movement, their foot catches, and they fall.

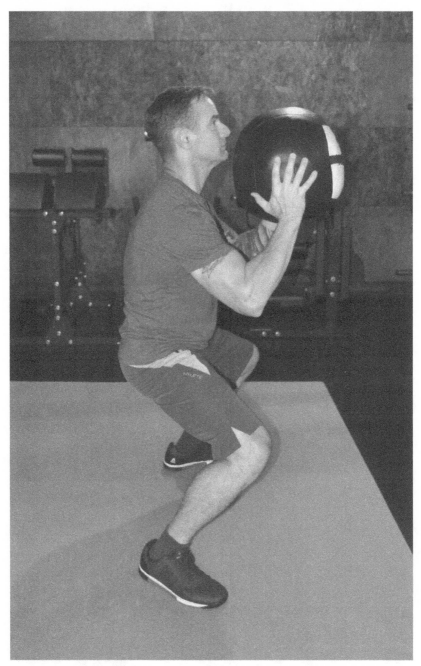

Figure 3.27.   Squat Throws

CHAPTER 3

Battle Ropes

Battle ropes are an excellent tool to add to your toolbox; however, battle ropes should be considered more as part of a complete workout as opposed to a complete workout in and of itself. Battle ropes can be done as either a low-intensity activity or high-intensity activity. It also can provide muscular endurance and plyometric work. The use of battle ropes involves the entire upper body for all exercises, and the lower body can be added during most of the movements. If you have the physical space to add in a set of battle ropes at home or if your gym has a set, I would suggest adding this to your program (see figure 3.28).

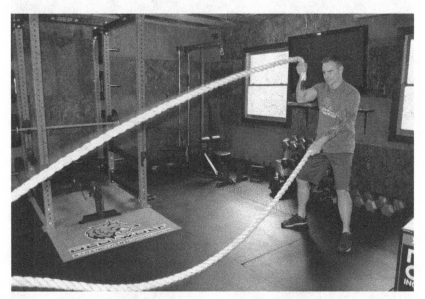

Figure 3.28.   Battle Ropes

4

DEVELOPING A
TRAINING PLAN

The previous chapters of this book discuss basic training principles, basic physiology, basic psychology, and areas of training for mixed martial arts (MMA). These chapters are important because they provide the necessary foundational information that will aid you in building a rock-solid training program. In this chapter, I provide information on how to develop a strong training program built around the demands of your everyday life.

When developing your program, there are a few key points to remember. The first is that more than one road exists, and there are many different paths to your destination. Do not get too caught up in designing the perfect program on your first attempt. Design a sound program, and make changes as you go based on marked improvements in performance and monitoring adaptation. Keep in mind that as long as you are not overtraining, you will be fine. Do not be afraid of making a mistake when developing your program, because you will. Just learn from those mistakes and improve. Understand that your strength and conditioning program is an evolving and learning process.

Another key point to remember is that you need to stick with your program design. While you do want the program to evolve with your progression, you do not want to move away from the key training principles, which are the foundation of program development. The key training principles will always remain true. One of the biggest mistakes beginners make is quitting a program before the training has an opportunity to elicit a positive change. They jump from program to program with no real gains. Develop a sound program, and stick with it. You will need to make alterations to volume and intensity based on how your body responds to the stimulus, but the program itself does not change.

Do not overload your program by trying to do too much. Another common mistake is to create a program that is too high in volume and intensity. Mixed martial artists want to be the strongest and fastest, and have the greatest endurance. So naturally, they put together a program that attempts to maximize every area at once. The problem is that many will take a program that optimizes strength improvements, another that optimizes power, and a third that optimizes endurance, and put them one on top of the other, resulting in an extremely high training volume that not even a professional fighter could handle. You are not training to be a powerlifter, Olympic lifter, or marathon runner. You are training to be a fighter. So develop a program that optimizes fighting performance.

Your technical skill and tactical training should remain the focus of your training, and strength and conditioning should be a supporting component. Never confuse the two. While a strength and conditioning program will make you a better fighter, it cannot take the place of your skill training, as that is the foundation of your martial arts program. Never rely on your strength and power, rely on your martial arts training and use your strength and power to complement your skill.

Start small and work your way up to the appropriate volume. Trying to do too much too soon will lead to overuse injuries and maladaptation. For example, if you have never used a strength or endurance program before, do not start with a full-blown program volume. Instead, add a little bit of each and work your way up to the desired and appropriate volume. Adding too much too soon can negatively impact your progression.

The last key point is to write everything down, as it avoids random, disorganized training. This is especially true when trying to work a training program into your everyday life. If you do not schedule and make your training a priority, things will get in the way and you will keep putting off your training until later and have no time to complete it. Take the time and effort to write out your program, as it provides a clear map to your desired goals. When you write down your training program, you are more likely to follow the plan. It is also a good idea to record your progression as well, as this allows you to track your short-term goals.

WORKING WITH A COACH

Second to yourself, your coach is the most important part of your training program. Most professional MMA athletes, at minimum, will have a skills coach and a strength and conditioning coach. In an ideal situation, a fighter would have a head coach, ground coach, stand-up coach, strength and conditioning coach, and sports nutritionist. These individuals work together to develop a training plan, monitor the training plan, monitor the athlete's response to training, and make the necessary adjustments. Unless you are a professional fighter, it is unlikely that you will have access to that level of training. It is more likely that you will have a skills coach and that you will have to act as your strength and conditioning coach, as well as your own sports nutritionist.

Just like with professional athletes, it is important that you coordinate with your skills coach when developing your training plan to optimize your progression. One of the biggest mistakes I see MMA athletes make is that they overtrain because they do not coordinate their strength and conditioning program with their skill training program. This is even more predominate when an MMA athlete participates in group martial arts training as opposed to individualized one-on-one sessions. Group martial arts classes are typically designed to improve both skill and conditioning within the same hour. If you put your strength and conditioning program on top of your MMA training with no adjustments to volume and intensity, it may be too much. This is especially true if your group MMA class does not use a methodological approach to conditioning. For clarity, there is absolutely nothing wrong with MMA group classes, and this is how most group classes need to be run to be successful for the majority of the students in the class; however, you must take this factor into consideration when developing your own program. For example, say you conducted interval training that morning as scheduled in your program and show up for your Muay Thai skills class that night, and the last 20 minutes of class is upper- and lower-pad striking burnouts. Both of these training sessions are important, and they have their place in your training schedule, but, in most cases, not on the same day. Keep in mind that high-intensity skill training under the observation of a skilled coach is absolutely necessary to improve performance in MMA.

The first approach to alleviate the issue of melding your skill training with your strength and conditioning is to pay for individual classes. This will allow you to better coordinate your strength and conditioning with your skill training for a well-rounded program. This will allow you to sit down with your coach and develop an optimal plan that provides a pathway to success. When you are able to plan your training with your coach, you will be able to see the process in its entirety.

If individual lessons are not available or viable, you will need to work your strength and conditioning program around your group classes. To accomplish this goal, you will need to make a schedule of your skill classes and the intensity of each class session. For example, if Wednesdays are sparring days, you will schedule Wednesdays as your high-intensity days. If every class is a high-intensity class, you will need to speak with your coach about going at a lower intensity and focusing on skill during specific classes. Do not be afraid to speak with your coach about needing to adjust your training.

Online Coaching

Online strength and conditioning coaching is another option that has become popular in recent history. With current technology, a coach can work with you online and never even meet with you face-to-face. Many modern watches contain GPS and heart rate monitoring, which allow coaches to evaluate performance, mark adaptations, and prescribe training based on those adaptations. Modern technology makes online coaching a viable option. Prior to committing to an online program, examine all coaching options, pricing, and reviews. While online coaching for strength and training is a viable option, it is not ideal for MMA skill training.

Online boxed training plans are another option you can use. These training plans provide a day-to-day generic training plan without the interaction of a coach. Boxed plans use a one-size-fits-all approach to training. There are no variations to these programs, as everyone receives the exact same program. You will receive a weekly training plan you can use to improve your performance, but you will receive no coaching or advice on how to alter the program to elicit optimal adaptations.

These rigid programs are designed so that the average person can increase performance while ensuring that overtraining does not occur. Typically, these programs provide lower volumes and intensities to prevent overtraining. Boxed training programs can be useful for beginners by providing a safe, structured place to begin training; however, if you want to excel in MMA, you will need to make adaptations to the training plan based on your progression and how your body is adapting to the training volume and intensity. If you are using one of these plans, it may be more difficult to fit into your technical training.

PERIODIZATION

Periodization breaks up the training cycle into specific training periods, allowing the athlete to optimize performance. The human body is not designed to continually adapt to high-intensity levels and volumes without recovery. In other words, you cannot train full speed year-round without allowing for recovery. By breaking your training into specific cycles, you can optimize both stimulus and recovery periods. The idea of periodization is to develop a training plan that allows the athlete to alter training intensity and volume to peak during the season with mini peaks throughout the season to optimize performance at key competitions. When looking at periodization you have three primary levels: macrocycle, mesocycle, and microcycle. First, we will discuss each level of periodization, and then I will provide example training plans.

Macrocycle

The largest of these cycles is called the macrocycle, and for most traditional sports it covers a year of training (preseason, season, and offseason). MMA arts differs from traditional sports in that there is no specifically defined time of the year that is considered the offseason, as fights occur throughout the year. The macrocycle for MMA can range anywhere from 10 weeks to a year depending on your individual goals. Individuals who are not interested or ready for competition will have a longer macrocycle, whereas those who want to compete in MMA will have multiple macrocycles within a year. There are numerous ways to use periodization to outline a successful program, but I will discuss two common scenarios and possible periodization options for MMA.

The first scenario I will discuss involves those who have scheduled fights for the upcoming year. To develop a macrocycle for the year, you will need to determine your fight schedule for that year. Typically, most professional MMA fighters only compete 2 to 6 times per year, while amateur fighters typically fight 15 or more times per year. The rationale behind only fighting 2 to 6 times per year is that your body needs time to recover from the damage sustained during a fight. Keep in mind that most organizations have required medical suspensions based on specific sustained injuries and will limit how frequently you can fight. When choosing your fights for the year you want to make sure you choose a realistic number and that they are spread out enough to allow recovery between fights. As an amateur, finding and scheduling fights can be difficult, and you may need to adjust your plans as your fight schedule changes. Ideally, you need at least a 10-week notice to adjust your training schedule to physiologically peak for your fight.

You will plan your macrocycle so that you peak for each of your chosen fights. If you are fighting twice a year, you will have two macrocycles, and if you are fighting four times per year, you will have four macrocycles. The more times you fight, the shorter the duration of each macrocycle. The macrocycle will last from the preparation phase to the transition phase of the mesocycle, discussed in the upcoming section.

The second scenario is for those individuals who wish to optimize their MMA performance but are not currently competing. If you fall into this category, you will want to develop your macrocycle in a yearlong program. This will allow you to appropriately vary your training throughout the year so you can optimize gains. Just like with those who have fights scheduled for the year, you will peak and transition multiple times throughout the year, with mesocycles (discussed later on this page) designed for improvement in specific areas. You can split up your year evenly into three macrocycles that are four months each or four macrocycles that are equally divided into three months each.

If you are a beginner who just started MMA training and would eventually like to fight, you will want to consider a quadrennial plan (a long-term, four-year plan). One of the biggest mistakes new fighters make is to fight too soon before they are ready. If you have no martial arts experience, you should expect at least one to two years before your first amateur fight. The time required before a first fight is highly variable and depends on how quickly an individual advances. A quadrennial plan will allow you to develop as a fighter during a four-year period in an organized, stepped approach. While you will not plan every training session for the four years in advance, you will pick specific goals to focus on during each year. Your long-term plan does not have to be four years; it can be two or three years as well.

Mesocycle

The mesocycle is a subcycle of the macrocycle and typically covers a four-week period of training. There are multiple phases that can be used within a mesocycle, which can alter depending on the specific goals of that cycle. Common phases in a mesocycle are preparation phase, build phase, peak/competition phase (taper occurs in this phase), recovery, and transition. Preparation phase is designed to increase volume, whereas the build phase increases intensity. It is important to always increase your volume prior to increasing your intensity. It is possible to slightly increase both as you progress; however, increasing intensity prior to volume could result in injury. It is often better to increase volume and then intensity.

The taper phase allows for active recovery leading into the fight. The taper allows you to make sure that your body is completely recovered and ready for the fight while not losing fitness. Oftentimes people mistakenly believe that you should drop your volume extremely low and do no intensity during the taper, but this methodology can be counterproductive. While volume will lower, you still want to maintain a base volume the week prior to the fight. You will also want to have a moderate-intensity day about five days out from the fight. The last two days prior to the fight should be low intensity and focus solely on skill. There will be no need for a taper phase if you are just peaking and not going into competition, as you will have a recovery phase after your peak instead.

The peak/competition phase is where you have peaked for that particular section of training. At this point, physiological gains should be optimized for that particular section of training. The peak period is a good time to measure progression to determine if your program is working correctly. You should see improvements in the areas that were the focus of that mesocycle. If you have peaked for competition, your performance during the fight will be the measure of your program effectiveness. Do not conduct physiological testing (VO_2 max, 1RM, etc.) prior to the fight, as most all physiological testing will put unwanted strain on your body.

After the peak/competition phase, you will need a short recovery period of lower volume and intensity before transitioning into the next phase. The recovery phase will focus on ensuring that the fighter recovers not only physically, but also mentally. As mentioned earlier, recovery will also be affected by any substantial injuries that occurred during the fight.

For an example of a mesocycle during a 13-week macrocycle for an individual who is planning to fight, see table 4.1.

Table 4.1. Example of a Mesocycle during a 13-Week Macrocycle for an Individual Who Is Planning to Fight

Weeks	1	2	3	4	5	6	7	8	9	10	11	12	13
Macro	Macro 1												
Meso	Preparatory			Build				Taper	Competition		Recovery	Transition	

Earlier we divided the year into three macrocycles for an individual who has no fights planned for that year. Table 4.2 is an example of a yearly mesocycle of one macrocycle for an individual who has no fights scheduled. This method allows you to go through a preparatory and build phase where you increase volume and then intensity during a 16-week period, which ends in a peak and transition. This allows you to continually build, hit the peak of that training schedule, recover during the transition phase, and then begin your second macrocycle of the year. This is important, as it allows you recovery periods throughout the year. ·

Table 4.2. Example of a Yearly Mesocycle of One Macrocycle for an Individual Who Has No Fights Scheduled

Weeks	1	2	3	4	5	6	7	8	9	10	11	12	13	14	15	16
Macro	Macro 1															
Meso	Preparatory						Build						Peak		Transition	

The focus of each mesocycle is highly dependent on the individual fighter. For example, if you have a fighter who needs to improve their cardiorespiratory fitness, you would focus on endurance training for a mesocycle. It does not mean that you would ignore other areas of training, but instead the training focus would be on increasing endurance performance. If you have a fighter whose ground technique is really good but they are often overpowered by individuals of the same weight class, you would want to focus on increasing strength and power. An example of a more focused mesocycle for improvements in strength and power appears in table 4.3.

Table 4.3. Example of a More Focused Mesocycle for Improvements in Strength and Power

Weeks	1	2	3	4	5	6	7	8	9	10	11	12	13	14	15	16
Macro	Macro 1															
Meso	Strength focus preparation			Strength focus build			Power focus preparation			Power focus build			Peak		Transition	

Microcycle

Now that you know the overall training goals (macrocycle) and have broken down those goals into purposeful training periods (mesocycle), the next step is to determine your weekly training schedule (microcycle). The microcycle is the weekly training program where you schedule day-to-day training. While a microcycle typically covers the entire week, you can break it down into smaller microcycles within a week's time period when needed.

When developing a microcycle for MMA, you will often need to schedule multiple types of training. For example, you will have MMA training and resistance training on the same day. The ideal way to accomplish this would be to conduct your MMA training and then go right into your resistance training; however, many people do not have a 2- to 2.5-hour block to train every day and may need to split it up into two training sessions (two-a-days). Another consideration is when you are able to train technical aspects with your coach. Oftentimes slots for training martial arts are limited. The first option is a more ideal situation in that you are able to complete your training in one session and have a long recovery period prior to your training session the following day. When conducting all of your training within one block of time, always complete your MMA training first. Conducting your strength and conditioning prior to MMA training will cause fatigue, resulting in poor skill performance. If you are conducting a two-a-day session, it is still ideal to conduct the MMA training first; however, if enough time has passed so that a morning session will not greatly impact a night MMA training session, you can conduct your strength and conditioning in the morning. As most martial arts lessons are taught at night, many people will need to conduct their strength and conditioning in the morning prior to work or during their lunch break.

I have set up the following microcycles with two recovery days (see tables 4.4, 4.5, and 4.6). There is an active recovery day on Wednesday, where you would just work on technique, with no conditioning, and a complete recovery day on Sunday. I set up Sunday as the complete recovery day due to martial arts classes typically being taught Monday through Friday only. But oftentimes an individual will have more time to train during the weekend. If that is the case, you can shift your days to the right by one day, where Monday becomes your recovery day. You can actually shift those days as many days as you like to fit your schedule.

PROGRAMMING

Now that you have a basic understanding of the macrocycle, mesocycle, and microcycle, you can use that knowledge to help you develop your training program. At this point you will be combining all the knowledge you have gained in the previous chapters to create a successful program. Be sure to reference earlier chapters as needed.

When developing your program, it is important to understand a few key factors that will allow you to better fine-tune your training and avoid major training mistakes. When developing your program, make sure to follow the basic FITT principle for determining frequency, intensity, time, and type of training. In the following sections I have reorganized the FITT principle into volume (composed of frequency and time), intensity, and type of training.

Table 4.4. Single Session

Day	Monday	Tuesday	Wednesday	Thursday	Friday	Saturday	Sunday
Training	MMA resistance*	MMA conditioning**	MMA	MMA resistance*	MMA	Conditioning**	Recovery

*Resistance can be muscular strength, muscular power, or muscular endurance training.
**Conditioning can be either cardiorespiratory endurance or anaerobic.

Table 4.5. Two-a-Days

Day	Monday	Tuesday	Wednesday	Thursday	Friday	Saturday	Sunday
Morning Training	Resistance	Conditioning		Resistance		Conditioning	Recovery
Evening Training	MMA	MMA	MMA (recovery intensity)	MMA	MMA		

Table 4.6. Two-a-Day Session with Combined MMA and Conditioning and MMA Recovery

Day	Monday	Tuesday	Wednesday	Thursday	Friday	Saturday	Sunday
Morning Training	Resistance			Resistance		MMA recovery*	Recovery
Evening Training	MMA	MMA conditioning	MMA	MMA	MMA conditioning		

*During MMA recovery work on form and strategy only. Intensity should be very low.

Volume

Your training volume will be made up of time and frequency. As stated earlier, frequency is how often you train. You will need to determine how many days per week you are able to devote to training. It is important to be realistic when determining frequency. I would love to conduct MMA training at my gym five days per week; however, I am married with four young boys (ages 9–14), coaching two days a week and working as a university professor, all of which keeps me very busy. So, instead of five days a week of MMA training at my gym, I do three days per week of MMA training at the gym and two more days of MMA training at home. You will need to determine what works best for you and your situation.

Scheduling two-a-day workouts needs to be done with care and careful consideration. The danger of two-a-day workouts is that they provide very little time for recovery and often result in overtraining when conducted incorrectly. The problem occurs when not enough time has passed to allow the body to fully recover and for energy stores to be replenished. Oftentimes fighters will go into the night training session fatigued from the morning session, train hard at the night session, and then wake up for the following morning session still not recovered. Your body must have time to recover from one day to the next to adapt optimally. This is why it is important to control the volume and intensity of both the morning and evening sessions. While it may sound as though I am against two-a-day training schedules, I am not. They can be used effectively if executed correctly. Due to the fact that I work during the day, I use a two-a-day training program where I use the morning session for conditioning and the night sessions for technique.

In previous chapters, I discuss numerous exercises for resistance training. Do not attempt to insert all of the exercises listed in this book into your training program at once, as the volume will be too high. The exercises are listed and explained in detail to allow you to choose those you want to implement into your program. These exercises are designed to achieve specific goals, and it is important to make sure that the exercises you choose are designed to align with your training goals for that particular phase. For example, you may want to increase your strength and conduct a phase of training to improve strength prior to starting your fight camp. Your strength phase will end prior to the beginning of your fight camp, and your fight-camp phase will begin. Each phase you choose will have specific goals, and your training should match those goals. It makes no sense to perform heavy lifting during your eight-week fight camp, when your main goal will be driving up your power and anaerobic threshold.

The length of each training session, which is determined by the number of exercises, intervals, and so on, will also make up your overall volume. Training sessions do not have to be long to be effective. Many of your individual training sessions will be less than an hour. Combined training sessions (MMA and resistance, MMA and conditioning, etc.) will typically be about two hours. If you have multiple regularly scheduled individual sessions that last longer than an hour, you need to evaluate your program and ensure that you are not overtraining. While you want to include travel time, changing time, social time, and so forth, into your daily time schedule, do not include those factors when evaluating training volume. Just include the time frame from the start to finish of your training session.

Volume of MMA training sessions can also be determined by number of strikes thrown during the session. These can be counted as they are thrown, via video analysis, or through a punch-tracking system (accelerometers). The first two methods work but are tedious. Punch-tracking systems are easy to use and provide instantaneous and cumulative data. The downside is that at the time of this publication, there are no systems that accurately track kicks, elbows, and knees.

Intensity

Intensity is another area that must be carefully considered when developing your program. Athletes have a tendency to attempt to go too hard too often, resulting in overtraining. Intensity should be monitored as closely as volume. You will need to alternate intensity (the hard–easy principle) throughout the week to optimize both stimulus and recovery. Monitor the intensity of your MMA sessions, as well as your strength and conditioning sessions. Too often every MMA session is turned into a high-intensity session. High-intensity MMA sessions are extremely important to your development and should be conducted as one of your hard conditioning days; however, not every MMA session needs to be a high-intensity session. Intensity will also shift through the cycles as the goal for each cycle changes.

As mentioned previously, you can monitor intensity for your endurance sessions using a heart rate monitor. A downloadable heart rate monitor will allow you to download data after the training session to look at overall intensity throughout the training session. A punch tracker can also be used to examine intensity, providing power readings for each punch thrown.

Type

The type of training that you choose will be highly dependent on the goal of that particular microcycle. As an MMA fighter can benefit from improvements in every training area, you will need to develop your program so that you can improve in those areas. You want to develop a toolbox that provides you with the tools to become the best fighter you can be. The toolbox has limited space; therefore, you must choose your tools wisely. The largest tool in the box should be your MMA technical training. The other tools that should go into the box are cardiorespiratory endurance, muscular strength, muscular power, muscular endurance, anaerobic capacity, flexibility, and nutrition. The size of these tools will vary by individual but will be smaller than tactical. They are all important, but they cannot all be trained to their individual maximal level. Remember that you are training to be the best fighter you can be and not the best runner, bodybuilder, powerlifter, and so on.

One of the common questions I receive is about the effect of concurrent training on increases in performance. Concurrent training is when you are conducting multiple types of training at the same time, for instance, strength and endurance training. Research has shown that concurrent training diminishes the individual effect of each type of training. In other words, if you are executing strength training and endurance training within the same program, you will not get as strong as you would if you were conducting strength training alone. You also would not see the gains in endurance performance that you typically would if you were conducting endurance performance alone; however, you will see moderate gains in both, which is fine for what you are trying to accomplish with your program.

Example Programs

In this section I provide outlines for the development of a basic program on the microcycle level with daily workouts. You will need to adjust these programs to fit your specific needs. Nonetheless, they will provide you with a good starting point. Moreover, keep in mind that you will need to build weekly microcycles that will address the specific sports performance goals of that period. It is beyond the focus (and page limit) of this book to write out every sequence of possible microcycles that someone would need.

The volume and intensity of your conditioning microcycle will be dependent on the goal of that particular mesocycle and microcycle, and your current fitness level. The focus of conditioning may be to increase cardiorespiratory fitness or

Table 4.7. Preparatory Phase with Focus on Increasing Volume

Day	Monday	Tuesday	Wednesday	Thursday	Friday	Saturday	Sunday
Morning Training	Resistance	:30 zone 2 running		Resistance		:45 zone 2 running	Recovery
Evening Training	MMA	MMA	MMA (recovery)	MMA	MMA		

Table 4.8. Build Phase with Focus on Increasing Anaerobic Capacity

Day	Monday	Tuesday	Wednesday	Thursday	Friday	Saturday	Sunday
Morning Training	Resistance	:30 zone 3 running		Resistance		:05 warm–up; 6 x 400 sprints; :01:45 pace; :05 cooldown	Recovery
Evening Training	MMA	MMA	MMA (recovery)	MMA	MMA		

anaerobic capacity, or a little of both. When looking at cardiorespiratory fitness, a recovery run for one fighter might be three miles, whereas that would be a moderate run for another fighter or even a long run for a beginning fighter. Tables 4.7 and 4.8 are examples of programming conditioning into your weekly training plan.

When working with muscular strength, muscular power, and muscular endurance, it is important to look at the overall volume (number of sets x number of repetitions) and intensity (weight). The volume of the workout will be highly dependent on your goals for that mesocycle and microcycle. You may not be concerned with strength gains during a specific mesocycle and instead are focused on increasing cardiorespiratory endurance and therefore choose a low-volume strength program for that mesocycle. Or you may be more concerned with increasing strength and therefore go with a higher-volume strength program and lower-volume cardiorespiratory program for that mesocycle. You may need to add exercises in as needed to address your individual needs. For example, if you have a muscular imbalance between your quadriceps (stronger) and hamstrings (weaker), you may want to add in leg curls to increase the strength of the hamstrings to offset the imbalance and reduce the risk of an ACL rupture. The following are examples of various workouts you can incorporate into your weekly program.

Table 4.9. Lower-Volume Strength Focus

Exercise	Sets	Repetitions
Bench press	3	4–6
Lat pulldowns or bent-over rows	3	4–6
Dead lifts	3	4–6

Table 4.10. Higher-Volume Strength Focus

Exercise	Sets	Repetitions
Bench press	3	4–6
Dumbbell press	3	4–6
Lat pulldowns	3	4–6
Seated rows	3	4–6
Squats	3	4–6
Dead lifts	3	4–6

Table 4.11. Muscular Endurance

Exercise	Sets	Repetitions
Push-ups	3	Assigned number* or volitional exhaustion
Dips	3	Assigned number* or volitional exhaustion
Pull-ups	3	Assigned number* or volitional exhaustion
Horizontal rows	3	Assigned number* or volitional exhaustion

*You will have an assigned number that falls in the range of muscular endurance (15-plus) or take each set to volitional exhaustion.

Table 4.12. Low-Volume Muscular Endurance and Muscular Strength

Exercise	Sets	Repetitions
Bench press	3	8–12
Lat pulldowns	3	8–12
Hip thrusters	3	8–12
Dead lifts	3	8–12

Table 4.13. High-Volume Muscular Endurance and Muscular Strength

Exercise	Sets	Repetitions
Bench press	3	8–12
Dumbbell press	3	8–12
Overhead press	3	8–12
Lat pulldowns	3	8–12
Seated rows	3	8–12
Hip thrusters	3	8–12
Squats	3	8–12
Dead lifts	3	8–12

Table 4.14. Muscular Power*

Exercise	Sets	Repetitions
Box jumps	3	10–15
Lateral box jumps	3	10–15
Squat throws	3	10–15
Chest passes	3	10–15
Overhead ball slams	3	10–15

*If you are familiar with power cleans or other lifts that improve muscular power, you can add them here.

Low-Volume Core

It is important to add in a core routine within your strength and conditioning program. Choose at least one core exercise that focuses on the muscles of the abdomen and one that focuses on the muscles of the back. When adding in core, your repetitions will be determined by an assigned number that falls in the range of muscular endurance (15-plus), or you will take each set to volitional exhaustion.

Do not forget to schedule in flexibility training when planning your microcycle. It is easy to ignore flexibility training, as it is often seen as a peripheral requirement and put off until later. Flexibility should be conducted both prior to and after all training sessions.

TRAINING LOG

Throughout the process of creating your training program it is vital that you put your plan into writing by developing a training log. The training log has multiple purposes that will assist you in your training and progression. The first purpose of a training log is to give you a detailed road map to follow. You will know exactly what the daily workout routine will be, and it will help keep you focused on your goal and prevent you from getting sidetracked.

The second benefit is that it will keep you motivated. Research has shown that if you write out your plans in detail, you are more likely to follow those plans. On days that you may not feel like working out, it will provide that little push to get you going. It helps with accountability.

The third major benefit is that recording your daily workouts allows you to monitor your progression. Improvements in performance occur slowly throughout time, and often we do not recognize these improvements. Looking back in your training log will allow you to assess your progression in a quantitative and detailed manner.

Developing Your Training Log

As your training log will be specific to your individualized program, it would be difficult to find a preprinted training log that would specifically fit your needs. Luckily with today's technology, creating your own training log with the specifics that you need is simple and affordable. I will provide key criteria you should use when developing your training log. Do not put so much information in your log that it becomes overwhelming and useless. You will need the following information when developing your log:

- *Date and time.* Record the date and time of the workout so you can reference patterns in your training and progression in the future.
- *Body weight and body fat percentage.* Tracking body weight serves two main purposes: It monitors alterations in body weight throughout time and tracks fluid loss when training in the heat to optimize rehydration. When possible, measure body weight before each training session and after a training session when training in the heat. Body fat percentage allows you to examine fat and fat-free mass during a period of time but does not need to be done every training session.
- *Morning heart rate.* Morning heart rate helps determine readiness for training. An increased morning heart rate during a span of consecutive days could indicate overtraining or dehydration. It also allows you to record adaptation to endurance training, as morning heart rate will decrease throughout time with training.
- *Type of training.* State the type of training conducted: MMA, resistance, plyometrics, and so forth. List the individual exercises if conducting resistance training.
- *Volume.* For cardiorespiratory training, record the distance and time of the session. For resistance training, you will want to record the sets and reps for each exercise. For anaerobic training, you will want to record the time, sets, and distances. The volume of MMA training sessions can be determined by time or number of strikes.
- *Intensity.* Record the intensity of the training session. Record all measures used to determine intensity during the training session. For resistance training, the weight will be the intensity, and heart rate or RPE will often be used for cardiorespiratory training. Also record time in and out of the desired training zone for cardiorespiratory training when appropriate. When conducting some forms of training, for example, sparring, you will want to give an RPE as opposed to heart rate, as the use of a heart rate monitor may not be practical.
- *General comments on the training session.* General comments provide an opportunity to include other pertinent information (weather, fatigue, injury, sleep, stress levels, etc.).

5

NUTRITION FOR
MIXED MARTIAL ARTS

O ne of the most important components of an athlete's training program is
nutrition. Too often athletes will spend a large amount of time developing
and implementing a training program but completely ignore any form of nutritional planning. It is important to develop a nutritional plan that will optimize
anabolic processes for recovery and provide adequate fuel for training and
competing. The purpose of this chapter is to provide a basic introduction to
nutrition to optimize mixed martial arts (MMA) performance. The guidelines
are general in nature and designed for healthy individuals who do not have dietary restrictions. If you are regularly taking medication or have a known illness,
check with your physician prior to altering your nutritional intake. If you have
dietary restrictions, it is always a good idea to work with a registered dietitian
who has a background in sports nutrition and can establish a detailed nutrition plan tailored to your specific needs and goals. Even if you have no dietary
restrictions, working with a registered dietitian with a background in sports
nutrition would be beneficial.

NUTRIENTS

There are six basic categories of nutrients that are important to understand
for athletic performance: carbohydrates, fats, proteins, vitamins, minerals, and
water. These nutrients are responsible for everything from energy transfer to
anabolic processes to heat regulation, and each plays a specific role in normal
body function. Having a basic functional understanding of the specific nutri-

ents, how each one works, where each nutrient originates from, and how each one impacts MMA performance will allow you to develop a rational and sustainable nutritional program.

Carbohydrates

Carbohydrates are one of the main fuel sources for the human body. Carbohydrates are ingested and converted into glucose for transportation in the blood and glycogen for storage in the muscles and liver. Glycogen is important as not only fuel for athletic performance, but also the only fuel source the central nervous system and brain can use for energy. When glycogen stores become low during prolonged exercise, you become fatigued and confused. This is typically termed *bonking* and is often experienced during long endurance performances. The human body is limited to roughly 2,000 to 2,500 kilocalories (kCals) of stored glycogen.

The daily recommended intake of carbohydrates will differ depending on volume of physical activity (athlete or nonathlete). For the nonathlete, about 50 percent of daily caloric intake should come from carbohydrates, whereas 60 to 70 percent of an athlete's daily intake should come from carbohydrates. To more precisely determine carbohydrate intake, the average individual should consume 5 to 6 grams (g) of carbohydrates per kilogram (kg) of body mass per day, and athletes should consume 7 to 10 grams of carbohydrates per kilogram of body mass per day. The range of 7 to 10 g/kg is highly dependent on the volume and intensity of training. As the training volume or intensity increases, so, too, will the recommended intake.

For example, a fighter weighing 74.83 kilograms (165 pounds) would need to ingest between 523.81 and 748.30 grams of carbohydrates each day, depending on training volume and intensity. To give you an idea of what that looks like in food, a cup of plain oatmeal contains about 28 grams of carbohydrates, a baked potato between 35 and 39 grams, and a small serving of pasta approximately 40 to 50 grams. As you can see, it will take some planning to replenish your carbohydrate stores on a heavy training day.

While the quantity of carbohydrate intake is a concern, so is the quality of carbohydrates ingested. Refined grains lose a significant amount of their nutrients during the refining process and should be avoided whenever possible. Whole grains, fruits, and vegetables are excellent sources of carbohydrates. Eliminate as many simple carbohydrates (simple sugars) from your diet as possible. Keep in mind that some simple carbohydrates are good, for instance, those found in fruit and milk; however, many simple sugars are not good, for example, those found in ice cream, soda, and candy. Instead focus more on complex carbohydrates (whole grains, vegetables, etc.).

The glycemic index measures the effect of carbohydrate ingestion on blood glucose levels. Foods that are below 50 on the glycemic index have little effect on blood glucose levels; however, foods that measure above 70 can cause a large increase in blood glucose levels, resulting in a significant spike in insulin (hyper-insulinemia), which in turn causes hypoglycemia (low blood sugar), resulting in fatigue. For this reason, it is recommended to stay away from foods that are high on the glycemic index. The one exception is during an extended training session lasting longer than an hour. Ingesting foods that are high on the glycemic index during a long training session will result in blood glucose spikes when you need them and in turn spare stored glycogen for later use.

Fats (Lipids)

Fats play many different roles in the body. They are used as a major source of energy, assist in thermoregulation, provide protection for vital organs, assist in the transport of fat-soluble vitamins, and aid in the production of hormones. Fats provide a major source of energy during prolonged endurance activities below anaerobic threshold. Once ingested, fats are stored as triacylglycerol in the body and provide a large amount of energy per molecule. The average individual stores approximately 70,000 to 80,000 kCals of fats in muscle and adipose tissue (around organs and just under the skin). Obviously, this number can vary from individual to individual.

There are several different categories of fats: saturated fats, unsaturated fats, and trans fats. Saturated fats can be found in such foods as meats, eggs, milk, and cheese. Unsaturated fats can be either monounsaturated (found in canola oil, sunflower oil, and almonds) or polyunsaturated (found in meat, eggs, nuts, fish, fruits, and vegetables). Trans fats are found naturally in small amounts in meats and dairy products and are not of great concern. Trans fat that are artificially made through hydrogenation are often found in processed foods and are very unhealthy. Trans fats that are made through hydrogenation are commonly found in such foods as cakes, snack foods, and fast foods.

Approximately 30 percent of your daily intake should consist of fats, with the majority coming from unsaturated fats. Less than 10 percent of your dietary intake should come from saturated fats. Stay away from trans fats, as they are detrimental to your health. Also stay away from extremely low-fat diets (<15 percent of daily intake), as they can have a strong negative impact on health and performance. Ingesting about 1 g/kg of body mass per day is ideal for most athletes.

Proteins

Proteins are primarily used for anabolic processes and provide limited energy during exercise. They are only relied on for energy production when glycogen stores are depleted. Proteins are vital in the recovery process, as they help rebuild tissue. Excess ingested proteins are not stored in the body and are converted to either triacylglycerol or glycogen for storage. Meat, seafood, poultry, milk, cheese, eggs, and nuts are primary sources of protein in the diet.

As an athlete, you should ingest 1.2 to 2.5 grams per kilogram of body mass each day. The amount of protein you need to ingest will be highly dependent on the volume and intensity of your training program. As volume or intensity increases, you will need to increase protein ingestion to support the necessary anabolic process that are required after training. It is important to note that taking in large amounts of protein can place a strain on the liver and result in dehydration and electrolyte imbalance; however, this is typically not a concern for healthy individuals who are not ingesting more than 4 grams per kilogram of body mass per day.

VITAMINS

Vitamins do not provide energy directly, but they are vital in many of the chemical processes that regularly occur in the human body. Here I give a few common examples. B vitamins and niacin are a significant part of the chemical process that ultimately results in the production of ATP; vitamin D is important for bone density; and vitamin C assists in iron absorption. There are many more examples of the role of vitamins in the body in relation to exercise and performance, and going through all of them is beyond the scope of this book. The key point is that vitamins are vital for both health and performance.

For most healthy fighters who maintain a well-balanced diet, there is no need to supplement with vitamins; however, for those who may not be eating an adequate diet, vitamin supplementation may be beneficial.

MINERALS

Calcium

Minerals are inorganic nutrients required for normal body function. The most abundant mineral in the human body is calcium, which plays a key role in many chemical processes in the body. Human bone mass consists of 60 to 70 percent calcium; therefore, it is crucial for maintaining a healthy bone density. Calcium is also stored in muscle and plays a major role in the chain of events that result in a muscle contraction. Calcium is primarily obtained by consuming dairy products.

Iron

Iron is another mineral that is necessary to maintain normal body function. Iron is used in the formation of hemoglobin and myoglobin. Iron is not required in large amounts and can easily be obtained through the ingestion of meat. Iron can also be found in plant sources like potatoes or beans; however, plants provide insufficient amounts of iron by themselves. Unless you are iron deficient or vegetarian, there is no real need to take iron supplements. Supplementing with too much iron can also have a negative health impact.

Iron-deficient anemia results from low iron levels in the body and presents as a feeling of fatigue due to a decrease in hemoglobin. Certain populations are at greater risk for the development of iron-deficient anemia. Female athletes are susceptible to the development of iron-deficient anemia due to iron loss occurring during the menstrual cycle, heavy sweating during training, and the high hemoglobin turnover rate associated with heavy training regimens. Vegetarians are also at risk due to the limited availability of iron in plants.

Phosphorus

Phosphorus is another mineral that is widely used in the body for various chemical processes. Phosphorus binds with calcium to form calcium phosphate, which is vital for bone growth and development. Phosphorus is also important for protein synthesis and responsible for the formation of ATP. Phosphorus is consumed easily in most diets and can be found in meats, dairy products, and cereals.

Electrolytes

There are three minerals that are considered electrolytes: chlorine, sodium, and potassium. Electrolytes are electrically charged ions that are found in the fluids of the body. It is important to keep electrolytes balanced in the body, as they help maintain homeostasis. Sodium and potassium are two electrolytes that athletes should be aware of when developing a sound nutrition plan. It is often stated that Americans ingest too much sodium in their diet, resulting in high blood pressure. While this is true and you do not want to take in excess sodium, athletes need to ingest greater amounts of sodium in relation to the average sedentary individual because of the excess sodium lost during training through sweat. The more you sweat, the more sodium you will lose. This is why ingestion of sodium after exercise in the heat is recommended and why many sports drinks contain sodium. This is also why pickle juice is recommended for reducing muscle cramps in the heat. It isn't actually the "pickle" portion of the juice that is beneficial; instead, it is the high concentration of sodium found in pickle juice.

Potassium also helps maintain homeostasis through electrical balance within the cells. Potassium is found in many common foods, for instance, bananas, citrus fruits, and potatoes. A small amount of potassium is also found in fish. Individuals who maintain a healthy diet will acquire sufficient potassium without supplementation.

WATER

Water is vital for both sustaining life and sport performance, as the human body is composed of approximately 60 to 70 percent water. Blood plasma consists of approximately 90 percent water and is responsible for the transportation of gasses, nutrients, and other compounds throughout the body. Blood plasma is also responsible for thermoregulation, as water is an excellent conductor of heat. When exercising it is important to develop and maintain a sound hydration plan.

During exercise, water is lost through sweating and respiration. As you sweat, water moves from the interstitial space and exits the body through eccrine sweat glands to evaporate on the skin and cool the body. Water from plasma will move from the blood vessels into the interstitial space to replace the lost water and equalize pressure between the blood vessels and interstitial space. This action results in an overall decrease in plasma volume and decreased ability to cool the body. Water loss during exercise can negatively impact both performance and health. Water loss that is equivalent to approximately a 2 percent decrease in body mass will negatively impact performance. As the water loss reaches a 5 percent decrease in body mass, there will be a negative impact on health. One of the primary health concerns with dehydration is the inability to properly thermoregulate, leading to heat-related illnesses.

Because of the high volume of fluid lost during prolonged exercise, the recommendations for average individuals (1.5 to 3 liters/day) cannot be applied to individuals who train on a regular basis. Thus, it is important to focus on replacing the volume of fluid that is lost during training or competition.

One of the best methods for determining water loss is to weigh yourself before and after your training session. It is important to weigh unclothed before and after so that you are not measuring the volume of water retained in your clothes after the training session. The difference in weight between your preexercise measures and postexercise measures represents the volume of fluid lost during the training session. The next step is to replace each pound lost with approximately 24 ounces of fluid. This rehydration recommendation assumes that you were properly hydrated prior to the exercise bout.

NUTRITION AND EXERCISE

To promote recovery, positive adaptations, and increased performance, you should spend some time developing a sound nutritional strategy. There are four basic areas to consider when developing a nutrition plan for exercise. The first is the type of nutrition—carbohydrates, lipids, proteins, and so on. The second involves the quality of nutrition. Choose high-quality foods. The third involves the volume, or caloric intake, of your nutrition plan. Finally, the fourth consideration deals with the timing of the meals.

Before Training or Competition

When examining precompetition/pretraining nutrition, timing, quantity, and type of nutrition must be addressed. Meals should be eaten two to four hours prior to competition. Eat light foods that will provide energy but do not take a prolonged period of time to digest. For example, slow-cooked oatmeal, bagels, or fruits make an excellent breakfast; however, you should probably avoid the sausage, egg, and cheese sandwich.

Training or competing on an empty stomach can negatively impact performance and possibly health, especially on high-intensity days. Not eating prior to a workout can lead to low blood glucose levels, resulting in feelings of fatigue and dizziness. There will be a larger effect at higher intensities due to an increased reliance on glycogen and glucose as a primary energy source. During high-intensity training, you will use almost 100 percent glucose and glycogen.

Low blood glucose levels occur most commonly in individuals who skip break-fast prior to their morning training.

It is also not recommended to eat a large meal just prior to a training bout or competition, as it will often leave you feeling sluggish and with gastrointestinal distress. During exercise, blood flow will be directed to areas that need it most, for example, the working muscles and the skin for cooling. It will also be redirected from areas that need it the least, for instance, the digestive tract. After eating a meal, blood is redirected to the digestive tract to properly digest the food. So, if a meal is eaten prior to exercise, these two systems are at odds. During exercise, inadequate blood flow will be redirected to the digestive system to properly digest a meal, leading to gastrointestinal distress.

As mentioned earlier, it is generally recommended to avoid most foods that are high on the glycemic index; however, ingesting carbohydrates that are high on the glycemic index just prior to the start of exercise will help spare glycogen during training sessions lasting longer than an hour. Carbohydrates high on the glycemic index will increase blood glucose levels fairly quickly, which in turn will spare glycogen stored in the liver. Carbohydrates, for example, sport gels, can be ingested approximately 5 to 10 minutes prior to the start of exercise. Supplementing with carbohydrates during a training session is only recommended for exercise lasting longer than an hour. Do not take in sport gels more than 10 minutes prior to the start of the event, as this could cause an early blood glucose spike, leading to an overshoot of insulin, low blood sugar levels, and fatigue.

During Training

During training sessions that last longer than an hour, you will need to take in carbohydrates. Glycogen stores are topped off at about 2,000 to 2,500 kCals in the human body and therefore become a limiting factor for energy production through glycolytic processes during prolonged exercise. Ingesting carbohydrates increases blood glucose levels and therefore spares glycogen stores in the liver, offsetting glycogen depletion and the resulting fatigue. Keep in mind that glycogen is used at a much faster rate during high-intensity exercise. Significant reduction in glycogen stores will never be a concern during a fight, as the longest fight you will compete in will take 29 minutes (five 5-minute rounds with one minute of recovery between rounds).

When training at high-intensity levels for longer than an hour, you should ingest 30 to 60 grams of carbohydrates every 45 to 60 minutes during exercise. This is also true for sessions occurring at lower intensities that last longer than an hour and a half. Choose carbohydrates that are easily digested and high on the glycemic index, as they will enter your system quickly. Energy gels and sports drinks are typical choices, as they provide both. In comparison, sports bars enter the system at a slower rate.

It is vital to remain hydrated during training and competition. This rule is even more crucial on hot, humid days, as you will lose a greater amount of fluid. Dehydration results in a decrease in performance and leads to heat-related illnesses. You can hydrate with water or a sports drink, or a combination of both. Hydrating with water during sessions lasting less than an hour and a half will be sufficient in most cases. High-intensity activities lasting an hour and a half could benefit from supplementing fluid intake with a sports drink. In training sessions lasting longer than an hour and a half, it would be beneficial to use a sports drink to provide hydration, electrolyte replacement, and carbohydrates.

If you start a fight fully hydrated, dehydration is not a major concern due to the short length of the fight; however, if you begin a fight dehydrated due to weight cutting, it can negatively impact both performance and health. Thus, it is vital that you begin every fight well hydrated. Keep in mind that this does not mean that you should not worry about fluid intake during a fight. Performance will decrease during the fight if you do not ingest fluids. Take in water before, during, and after the fight.

It is difficult to completely maintain hydration levels during a long training session in the heat; therefore, it is vital that you develop a hydration plan and stick with it throughout the training session. Thirst is a mechanism that lets us know that dehydration is setting in and that we need to drink. During exercise, if you wait until you are thirsty to drink, it is already too late; you have already begun a downward spiral that can lead to decreased performance and the development of heat-related illness.

After Training and Competition

Recovery is an important component of any training program, and nutrition is key in the recovery process. What you ingest after a workout is just as important as what you take in before and during a workout. Training applies the necessary stress for positive adaptations and eventual performance increases to occur; however, this stress results in catabolic responses during exercise. It is the anabolic process, which occurs after exercise, that ultimately results in improved performance. Postexercise recovery not only helps with the anabolic processes, but also begins the refueling process.

You must start refueling within 1 to 2 hours after the completion of exercise. The typical recommendation to optimize recovery is within 45 to 60 minutes.

The four primary nutrients to ingest are water, electrolytes, carbohydrates, and proteins. Replace each pound of fluid lost through sweating with approximately 24 ounces of fluid. Use of a sports drink can be beneficial for both fluid and electrolyte replacement.

Carbohydrates and proteins should be ingested using a 4:1 ratio (4 grams of carbohydrates to 1 of gram proteins). Carbohydrates are necessary for replenishing glycogen stores, and proteins are vital for supporting the anabolic processes after exercise. You cannot completely replenish glycogen stores right after a workout; it will be an ongoing process throughout the rest of the day. Ingesting protein after exercise also assists in glucose and amino acid uptake into the muscles; moreover, it influences insulin levels. These factors are why the 4:1 ratio has been so successful during the recovery process. Recovery sports drink mixes that provide the necessary 4:1 ratio have been shown to be very effective at aiding recovery. Research has demonstrated that chocolate milk provides the same ratio and the same benefits.

BODY COMPOSITION

Body composition is the portions of the body in relation to fat and fat-free mass (muscle, bone, tissue, etc.). One of the most accurate and commonly used methods for determining body composition is body fat percentage, which examines the percentage of fat-to-fat-free mass. For example, a body fat recording of 15 percent indicates that the individual's body mass is 15 percent fat and 85 percent fat-free mass. Monitoring body fat percentage is an excellent way to track changes in your body composition.

For General Health

Many people begin martial arts for health reasons and the desire to get into better shape. In the United States, more than 65 percent of people are classified as overweight, and more than 30 percent are classified as obese. Being overweight or obese can result in various negative health conditions, including hypertension, high cholesterol (LDL) levels, type II diabetes, cardiovascular disease, certain types of cancer, gallbladder disease, joint problems, breathing problems, and all-cause mortality. Keep in mind that overweight individuals who are physically active are less likely to develop cardiovascular disease in relation to individuals who are thin but sedentary.

If you are participating in martial arts for health reasons or because you enjoy the activity, you need not worry too much about body composition. By training and eating right, body composition will take care of itself throughout time. The recommended body fat percentage range is 8 to 19 percent for males and 17 to 28 percent for females. Maintaining a healthy body composition within these recommended ranges is ideal for promoting optimal health. Classification of overweight begins at a body fat percentage greater than 20 percent for men and 30 percent for women. As body fat percentage increases beyond the initial classification of overweight, health risk increases significantly. Remember that having too little body fat can also have a negative impact on health. The essential body fat percentage for normal bodily functions is 4 percent for males and 12 percent for females.

For Competition

If you wish to truly compete in MMA, you will need to be a little more concerned with body composition due to weight class. Fighters are divided into weight classes to focus more on skill and less on size and strength advantages. Given that your opponent will be in the same weight class, having a greater lean body mass in relation to your overall body mass will give you a physical advantage during a fight. For instance, if you have two fighters that weigh in at 180 pounds and one fighter has 4 percent body fat while the other fighter has 12 percent body fat, it is evident that the fighter at 4 percent body fat will have a distinctive strength advantage. From this example, you can see how body composition plays an important role in combat sports. In this section I will focus on long-term weight management and not on weight cutting for a fight. I will discuss weight cutting a little later in chapter 6.

The recommended ranges for body compositions for competitive fighters are 4 to 10 percent for males and 12 to 20 percent for females. The reason there is such a wide range is that there will always be individual variability in body composition and, in general, there is an increase in body fat percentage as weight classes increase. While a low body fat percentage may be desirable for competition, there are a few factors that you must consider. The first is that a low body fat composition is very difficult to achieve and maintain. The closer an athlete gets to the lower end of the recommended athletic range, the greater the risk of decreased performance and compromised health. The second consideration is that not everyone will respond in the same manner to decreased body fat percentages. I have worked with elite-level athletes whose performance dropped when their body fat percentage became too low, even though it was above the recommendations for an elite-level athlete. If your body fat percentage drops into the lower range, you will need to make sure you carefully monitor both performance and health. The goal is to be as light as possible without negatively impacting health or performance.

Measuring Body Composition

If you are serious about performance, you will want to track changes in body composition throughout time. Different methods for determining body composition are described in this section, along with the advantages and disadvantages of each. You will want to choose a method that is both accurate and feasible.

Body Mass Index

Body mass index (BMI) is solely based on height and weight. BMI provides a simple and easy way to determine if an individual is underweight, normal, overweight, or obese. BMI can be calculated using either the metric or English/imperial system. Formulas for both systems are provided here. Once you calculate your BMI, you can then refer to the chart to determine which category you fall into.

English
$$BMI = 703 \times \text{weight (pounds)} \div \text{height}^2 \text{ (inches}^2)$$

Metric
$$BMI = \text{weight (kg)} \div \text{height}^2 \text{ (M}^2)$$

Once you have calculated your BMI, you will need to determine the range your calculated number falls into. If your BMI is <18.5, you are considered underweight. Normal BMI falls between 18.5 and 24.9, overweight is considered to be between 25 and 29.9, and obese is classified as a BMI ≥30.

BMI is an excellent tool for estimating body composition for large-scale populations, but it loses validity when examining individual athletes. The reason that BMI is not very useful when working with athletes is the fact that muscle is denser than fat and therefore weighs more. At the time of this publication, I weighed 194 pounds, and my height was 71.75 inches. This would make my BMI 26.49, classifying me as overweight; however, my body fat is at 8 percent and thus would not be classified as overweight. This demonstrates the primary disadvantage of relying on BMI to determine body composition when working with athletes.

Bioelectrical Impedance

Bioelectrical impedance systems use electrical currents to estimate body fat percentage. These systems require that you make contact with either the hands or feet. Once contact is made, the system passes an electrical current through the body to measure resistance to flow. Lean body tissue contains high concentrations of water; therefore, the electrical current passes through the body easily. Fat contains little water and hence provides resistance to flow. As fat stores increase, resistance to flow also increases. It is a fast and easy method for determining body composition. But bioelectrical impedance systems are neither reliable nor accurate.

Bioelectrical impedance systems rely heavily on the ability of the electrical current to easily flow through water. Thus, hydration levels significantly impact body fat percentage estimates. Your hydration levels during training will continuously fluctuate, especially in the hotter months, resulting in large fluctuations of bioelectrical impedance readings. Due to the large fluctuations in hydration levels and the inherent variability in these machines, I do not recommend them for measuring body composition.

Hydrostatic Weighing

Hydrostatic weighing (underwater weighing) has long been considered the gold standard for determining body composition. This method is based on Archimedes' principle, which states that the weight of water displaced by the body is equivalent to the buoyant forces acting on that body. Lean body mass (muscles, bones, organs, etc.) has greater density than water and therefore sinks, and fat is less dense than water and therefore floats. The amount of lean mass and fat mass will determine how buoyant an individual is in water.

While hydrostatic weighing is considered the gold standard, the process requires large, specialized equipment and trained professionals to conduct. This method requires the use of a water tank large enough for a human to completely submerge themselves underwater without touching the sides or bottom of the tank. The athlete must also be able to completely submerge, exhale as much air as possible, and remain still long enough to obtain a steady measure of underwater weight. This process makes it difficult for those who are uncomfortable underwater.

Dual-Energy X-Ray Absorptiometry

Dual-energy x-ray absorptiometry (DXA) determines body composition through the use of two low-energy x-ray beams and has the ability to accurately measure density and distinguish between fat and fat-free mass. Due to this method's accuracy and reliability, it is often considered the best way to determine body composition; however, the DXA system is extremely expensive and requires specialized skill to operate.

Calipers

Of all the methods mentioned, I recommend the use of skinfold calipers for determining body composition. Skinfold calipers are accurate, inexpensive, easy to use, and far more accessible and affordable in relation to other methods. Skinfold calipers work by pinching a fold of skin and fat, and measuring the thickness of the fold. From the skinfold measurements, total fat stores are estimated using simple formulas. Skinfold calipers cost anywhere from $25 to $200. The major differences between a lower- and a higher-cost caliper is the accuracy and durability.

Conducting skinfold testing is relatively simple but does take some practice to master. There are different tests used to measure skinfolds, but the three-site test is the one that is most widely used. The most common sites used for men are the chest, abdomen, and thigh. The three most common sites for females are the triceps, iliac, and thigh.

When conducting skinfold measures, it is important to accurately measure each site as described. Position the hand so that the fingers point down, and fold the skin between the thumb and index finger, as shown in figure 5.1. Once your fingers are positioned over the correct spot, pinch the skin, bringing it up into a fold. For an accurate measurement, pinch skin and fat only. Too large a pinch typically results in getting muscle, which results in an inaccurate measurement. Next, place the caliper pincers directly below your thumb and index finger with the gauge facing up so that you can read it. Once the caliper is in position, allow the calipers to close on the fold by slowly releasing the lever. Do not release the skinfold with your fingers until you record the measurement and remove the calipers. If you release the skinfold prior to the calipers, it can be slightly painful. Take three to four measurements at each site to ensure consistent readings. It is important to measure precisely in the locations described to obtain valid measurements. It is also important to be consistent with your measurements.

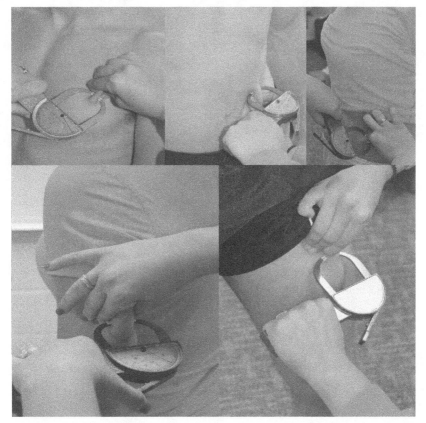

Figure 5.1. Skinfold Sites

The following instructions will provide you the necessary information to conduct a simple three-site test.

Chest: The chest is located along the outer edge of the pectoralis major at the midpoint of the muscle. The skinfold should be in line with the outer edge of the muscle.

Abdomen: The abdomen is located in line with the navel and one inch toward the side. Fold the skin vertically, not horizontally.

Iliac: The iliac is located just above the hip bone. Fold the skin in line with the natural crease at the hip bone.

Triceps: The triceps are located at the back of the arm, centered and halfway between the shoulder and elbow. Fold the skin vertically.

Thigh: The thigh is located on the centerline of the thigh halfway between the hip and patella. Fold the skin vertically. When working with athletic women it can be difficult to properly obtain the correct measurements. As the thigh is a primary storage location for fat in women and athletic women have significant muscle mass in the legs, it may take a harder pinch to accurately measure.

Once you have recorded all three sites, take the sum of the readings and plug the necessary data into the following equations:

Men
Body density = 1.10938 – (.0008267 × sum of skinfolds) + (.0000016 × [sum of skinfolds]^2) – (.0002574 x age)

Women
Body density = 1.0994921 – (.0009929 × sum of skinfolds) + (.0000023 × [sum of skinfolds]^2) – (.0001392 × age)

This first step gives you the estimated body density for the three-site skinfold test. Once body density has been established, the next step is to determine body fat percentage using the following formula:

Body fat percentage = (4.95 ÷ body density) – 4.50 × 100

Example Equation
Male: age = 25, chest = 5, abdominal = 9, thigh = 4 (total = 18)
Body density = 1.10938 – (.0008267 × 18) + (.0000016 x [18]^2) – (.0002574 × 25)
Body density = 1.088
Body fat percentage = (4.95 ÷1.088) – 4.50 × 100 = 4.96 percent

WEIGHT MANAGEMENT

Whether your weight management goal is for weight loss, health, or competition, there are a few important concepts you should keep in mind. The first and foremost is patience. No one puts on excess weight overnight; therefore, it is unrealistic to believe you can lose it overnight. Remain patient, avoid undue frustration, and stick with the plan. It is common to become frustrated with your progression. When things get frustrating, ask yourself, "Do I want to be standing here a year from now having lost weight or do I want to be standing here a year from now saying I wish I would have stuck with it and lost weight?" An important tool to help eliminate frustration is tracking your weight loss throughout time. It is important to note that weight fluctuates from day to day. Do not let this phenomenon discourage you from your ultimate goal.

Second, recognize that weight loss is not an easy process. You must be prepared for hard, physical work to achieve your goal. Additionally, you will need to implement a safe and healthy diet to accomplish your goal. Ignoring these simple facts will result in frustration and failure.

Lastly, it is important to understand that not everyone responds to weight loss in the same manner. Do not compare your weight loss to that of someone else. This is unrealistic and counterproductive; however, it does not mean that you cannot work in a group toward the same goal. Working with a support group can be very beneficial. Just do not compare your journey with that of other members of the group.

Factors That Affect Weight Management

Genetics

Genetics play a major role when it comes to body composition. Research shows that children of overweight parents are much more likely to be overweight than children of non-overweight parents. The distribution of body fat in the body is also strongly affected by genetics. It is easier for some people to lose weight, while others continuously struggle, but this does not mean that you are fated to be overweight just because you have a genetic predisposition to weight gain. It simply means that you need to be more careful of how you eat and how much exercise you get on a regular basis.

Lifestyle

While genetics is one of the key factors in determining body composition, lifestyle choices have the largest effect on body composition. Lifestyle is defined as the daily choices you make that affect how you live your life. The two key lifestyle choices that affect body composition are physical activity and diet.

Eating out often is one of the common mistakes people make. Food offered at sit-down and fast-food restaurants typically contains more calories in one meal than most people need in one day. At this point, I am only focusing on the caloric content and not the nutritional value of the food. Also, keep in mind that this is a generic statement that covers the vast majority of restaurants; there are restaurants that provide good portion sizes and healthy options.

It would be unrealistic to never eat out or grab something from a takeout restaurant. The following are a few guidelines that can help you when you do choose to eat out. The first recommendation requires a little preplanning on your part. Determine the caloric content of the foods that are offered at the restaurant you plan on visiting. Many restaurants provide this information on their online menu.

Another option is to decrease your portion size. Many restaurants will have different options when it comes to portion size, which allows you to order the portion size that best suits your needs. If there is only one option for portion size and it is too large for you, simply do not eat it all. Just because you order the meal does not mean you have to eat all of it in one sitting. Too often I have ordered a meal, eaten the entire thing, and then felt miserable afterward. One way to avoid this scenario is to portion your meal when you receive it, only eat the prescribed portion, and take the rest home for another meal. If you do not have the willpower to stop eating when you are full, ask for a "to go" box at the beginning of the meal and place the portion that you do not plan to eat in the box to take home. If you are eating with someone who has similar taste, you can also consider sharing a meal.

Preparing and eating meals at home, if done correctly, is the best option when it comes to managing body composition. Ideally, you want to prepare meals from fresh foods that are not excessively processed. Eating healthy is not as expensive as one might think, and you will discover that it is much less expensive in relation to eating out. Another misconception is that you have to spend hours in the kitchen to cook healthy meals. While the time to cook a meal does vary, depending on what you are cooking, there are many healthy meals that can be prepared quickly. If you are not familiar with healthy cooking, consider buying a cookbook that focuses on the subject. You will find healthy, tasty meals that are easy to prepare.

Even when eating healthy at home, you need to be aware of portion sizes. Modern dishware has gotten larger throughout time, and if you fill your plate you will probably take in more calories than you need. Most of us were raised on "cleaning" your plate before leaving the table so as to not waste food. While the logic behind this practice is understandable, it is much better to listen to your stomach and stop eating when you are full.

Meal planning is one method that will save you time and effort, and allow for healthy meals. The first step to eating healthy begins when you make your grocery list. Making a healthy grocery list and sticking to that list will help eliminate unhealthy eating. This helps prevent those impulse buys when you walk past an item that looks appetizing. If you do not buy junk food, you can't eat junk food. It is also not a good idea to grocery shop after a hard workout when you are tired and hungry. Whenever I shop hungry, my grocery basket always seems to be fuller and filled with some less-than-healthy choices.

Always read the nutrition label when purchasing foods to determine cholesterol, sodium, sugar, total calories, and so forth. When examining the caloric content, it is important to determine how many calories per serving, as well as serving size. For example, a serving size may be a half cup and a caloric content of 80 calories per serving. If you ingest a full cup, then the caloric content would be 160 calories.

Another valuable tool for weight management is a nutritional log. Keeping a nutritional log of everything you eat for the day will allow you to determine the volume of calories ingested each day. This is an eye-opener for many individuals, as they do not realize how many calories they ingest in a single day. This is an effective tool for demonstrating the need for a change in lifestyle. When keeping a nutritional log, record everything that you ingest and the calorie content of each. Keep in mind that this includes everything you eat, including snacks and everything you drink. Keeping a nutritional log is tedious work and may not be something you want to maintain on a permanent basis, but try to keep a log until you have made the proper adjustments to your eating habits.

Goals for Weight Management

Setting goals for your weight management program is an important part of the process. Weight loss will be challenging for everyone; therefore, it is important that you set realistic long-term and short-term goals. Setting a weight loss goal of 10 pounds in an 8- to 10-week period would be realistic for most individuals, whereas setting a goal of losing 10 pounds in a week would be very unrealistic. Setting unrealistic goals will negatively impact your weight management program and lead to serious discouragement. As mentioned previously, losing weight takes a long period of time, and you must remain patient. Setting short-term goals in conjunction with your long-term goal will allow you to monitor small steps in progression throughout time and help limit discouragement.

Safe, effective, and sustainable weight loss is considered to be roughly a loss of one pound per week. There will be weeks where you lose more and others where you lose less. Understand that weight will fluctuate, and do not become discouraged.

To optimally set weight management goals you will need to know your current body composition, as well as your desired body composition. The first step in this process is to determine your current body weight and body fat percentage, discussed earlier in this chapter. The next step is to determine your desired body composition. While most elite-level fighters have very low body fat percentages (males as low as 4 percent and females as low as 11 percent), this is an unrealistic goal for many. For many people, the goal of 8 to 19 percent for males and 17 to 28 percent for females is a good and achievable goal. I understand that I have provided a wide range of body fat percentages for both male and female fighters; however, where you would like to be in that range is a personal choice and completely up to you. Once you have determined your current weight, current body fat percentage, and desired body fat percentage, use the following formulas to determine weight loss:

(Current weight) × (current body fat percentage) = weight of fat in the body
Current weight – weight of fat in the body = weight of fat-free mass
1 – desired body fat percentage = percent fat-free mass
Weight of fat-free mass ÷ percent fat-free mass = desired body weight
Current body weight – desired body weight = desired weight loss

Example
Male: 210 pounds, currently 22 percent body fat, desires 12 percent body fat
(210 pounds) × (.22) = 46.2 pounds
210 pounds – 46.2 pounds = 163.8 pounds
1 – .12 = .88
163.8 pounds ÷ .88 = 186.14 pounds
210 pounds – 186.14 pounds = 23.86 pounds

In this example, a 210-pound male with a body fat percentage of 22 was able to determine that his desired body weight would be 186.14 pounds and that he would need to lose 23.86 pounds to reach the goal of 10 percent body fat. Remember, the goal is really about body composition and not weight. As muscle is denser in relation to fat, it weighs more. As you train, muscle will hypertrophy throughout time and increase the weight of your lean body mass; therefore, you will need to periodically rework the equations and adjust your weight management goals.

Caloric Balance

In its most simplistic form, weight management is all about caloric balance. When your caloric consumption is equivalent to your caloric expenditure, your body composition will remain at a near-constant. If you consume more calories than you expend, you will gain weight. If you consume less calories than you expend, weight will decrease throughout time. It would be extremely difficult to count the precise number of calories consumed and expended during a single day; however, counting calories in and calories out as precisely as possible will give you a good starting point. Some days you will take in slightly more than you use, and others you will take in slightly less than you use. But an overall deficit will balance out throughout time, resulting in weight loss. Keep in mind that if caloric intake remains too low for too long, metabolism can decrease, which is counterproductive to weight management. Extremely low caloric intake can also lead to catabolism of lean tissue, primarily muscle, in the body, which is also counterproductive.

It is commonly recommended that males take in between 2,000 and 2,500 calories per day and females between 1,500 and 1,800 calories per day. It is important to keep in mind that these recommendations are for the average male and female who do not participate in regular athletic training and therefore would represent insufficient calories for most fighters. A typical hour-long training class for MMA can burn anywhere from 300 to 600 calories depending on intensity and type of training. To optimally determine caloric requirements, you must first estimate how much you use on any given day.

The first step in determining caloric balance is to measure basal metabolic rate (BMR) or resting metabolic rate (RMR), which is the minimum energy required to properly maintain normal body function at rest. Both BMR and RMR will provide similar numbers and differ only in methodology of measurement. Resting metabolic rate typically provides numbers that are slightly higher than BMR, but the terms are often used interchangeably. For the purpose of this book and to eliminate confusion, I will use the term *basal metabolic rate*. Basal metabolic rate generally ranges from about 1,100 kCals to 2,100 kCals/day. It is the minimum energy required just to exist, and any physical activity conducted throughout the day will add to BMR. This is why the typical daily caloric recommendations for individuals range from 1,600 kCals/day for females to 2,500 kCals/day for males. These numbers go up for physically active males and females.

A linear relationship exists between heart rate and increased metabolism (typically estimated by VO_2); therefore, heart rate can be used to estimate BMR.

To estimate BMR using heart rate, you will need a heart rate monitor that estimates kCals at rest. Record caloric expenditure at rest for 10 minutes and mul-
tiply by 6 to determine caloric expenditure for an hour. The resultant number is
then multiplied by 24 to determine caloric expenditure for an entire day (BMR).

Laboratory testing for BMR and RMR is time consuming and expensive.
Thus, formulas are often used to estimate both. While formulas are not as accurate as direct measures, they can provide a fairly arcuate estimation and a great
place to begin.

Male
kCals/day = 66 + (13.7 × body weight in kg) + (5 × height in cm) – (6.9 × age)

Female
kCals/day = 665 + (9.6 × body weight in kg) + (1.7 × height in cm) – (4.7 × age)

Example Problem
Male, 180 pounds (81.63 kg), 72 inches tall (182.88 cm), age 25
kCals/day = 66 + (13.7 × 81.63) + (5 × 182.88) – (6.9 × 25) = 1,926.23 kCals

After BMR has been determined, caloric expenditure due to activity will
need to be added to the equation. If you had a morning run that used 600
kCals and then went for a short hike with your kids and used 200 kCals, you
would then add those 800 kCals to your BMR. Any physical activity (mowing
the lawn, cleaning the house, etc.) above resting needs to be added on top of
BMR. Keep in mind that this methodology is not 100 percent accurate and only
gives you a ballpark number. This is why counting calories ingested, counting
calories used, and measuring changes in body mass are important components
of weight management. If you lose or gain too much weight, you need to adjust
caloric intake accordingly.

Most heart rate monitors can estimate energy expenditure for endurance activities based on heart rate. The estimations provided by most heart rate monitors will be decently accurate for endurance activities, but heart rate monitors
cannot provide an accurate estimation of caloric expenditure for such activities
as interval training or resistance training. For these activities, you can use metabolic equivalents (METs) to help determine energy expenditure for specific
activities. One MET is equal to 3.5 ml/kg/min, which represents a resting state.
So, each MET you go above one is an activity level above your resting state.

The first thing to determine when using METs to calculate energy expenditure is the particular METs for the activity you are conducting. If you are lifting

weights the METs will range from 3 (very light) to 6 (vigorous). You will need to determine where your overall intensity was for that session. An example of a 3 would be when you first start lifting and you are working on technique, not pushing a lot of weight, and stopping at a set number of reps before volitional exhaustion. An example of a 6 would be when you are lifting at high intensity to volitional exhaustion with each set. The metabolic equivalent for sparring would be between 8 and 13 METs, a heavy bag workout between 7 and 10 METs, a technique class between 6 and 10 METs, and jiujitsu between 8 and 14 METs. This is a wide range of METs for each of those activities, and you will need to determine the intensity for each of your individual sessions.

You can also use METs to estimate energy expenditure for endurance activities. You can find the METs for running at any given speed. For example, the METs for running at a 12-minute-per-mile pace would be about 8 METs, and a 6-minute-per-mile pace would be about 15 METs. Be careful when using METs based on minute-per-mile pace, as you could be running an average 10-minute-per-mile pace because you are running a hilly course. Your speed of running will not always measure intensity or energy expenditure.

To calculate energy expenditure from METs, you will need your current body mass in kilograms, the time spent conducting the activity, and the METs for that activity. When looking at time for running it is fairly simple; know your start and stop time. When looking at something like a resistance training session it is not as straightforward. If you go in and conduct your resistance training and stay on task, you can count your entire session as time. If you go in and spend a lot of time talking and extend an hour-long session into a session lasting an hour and a half, you only count the hour. Keep in mind that these are estimations, but you want to be as accurate as possible. The following is the formula and an example problem:

(METs)(body mass in kilograms)/60 = kCals/min
An 81.63-kilogram male athlete conducted 45 minutes of sparring at a vigorous intensity.
(13 METs)(81.63 kg)/60 = 17.69 kCals/min
(17.69 kCals/min)(45 min) = 796.05 kCals

As you can see in this example, this individual's caloric expenditure for the sparring session would be 796.05 kCals. I used the same numbers from the earlier example where I calculated BMR. So, at this point in the day this individual would have expended 2,722.28 kCals (BMR of 1,926.23 kCals plus a sparring session of 796.05 kCals). You would add in any other significant energy expenditure throughout the day to get a total for the day. Next subtract energy consumed during the day to determine your net caloric balance.

When training for MMA, make sure to replenish the calories used throughout the day. This process is vital for energy replenishment, as well as for driving anabolic processes for recovery. As mentioned previously, it is all about manipulating caloric balance to reach your specific weight management goals. If you know how many calories you burned throughout the day, you know how many you need to replace. This is where your nutrition log can be helpful. By reading the caloric content of the food you consume and keeping track of the totals, you can compare caloric expenditure to caloric intake. Keep in mind that it is not only about the volume of nutrients, but also the quality of the nutrients.

Fad Diets

One of the biggest mistakes people make in the pursuit of their desired body mass is looking for shortcuts. Unfortunately, there are no safe or sustainable shortcuts to weight management. This tendency for individuals to look for the fastest and easiest way to lose weight has resulted in a market for fad diets. There is no short, fast, easy, or magical way to weight loss. Weight loss is a long and gradual process that requires dedication and work. Stay away from fad diets— they do not work. When it comes to weight loss, if it seems too good to be true, it is. Fad diet programs result in no change in body composition at best and lead to health-related problems at worst.

In recent history, low-carbohydrate and no-carbohydrate diets have been pushed as a healthy and fast way to lose weight; however, there is nothing healthy about a low-carb or no-carb diet. This is doubly true for an athlete. There are three primary reasons to stay away from a low-carb diet. The first and foremost is that the only source of fuel the central nervous system and brain can use is glycogen (the storage form of carbohydrates). Inadequate supplies of glycogen result in mental confusion and fatigue. As a survival mechanism, the body will produce glycogen by breaking down protein in the body. Excess protein is not stored in the body; therefore, muscle is degraded to provide the protein required for conversion to glycogen.

Use of lipids as a fuel will also be compromised due to low glycogen stores. As stated earlier in the book, lipids require glycogen to be completely catabolized for energy. Low glycogen stores and compromised lipid catabolism results in a decrease in pH (increased acidity). Other common complications of a low-carb diet are dehydration, electrolyte imbalance, strain on the liver, strain on the kidneys, consistent fatigue, and decreased cognitive function.

A low-carbohydrate diet will negatively impact both training and performance. Glycogen stores are extremely important when training or racing at high intensities. Because glycogen stores are limited to approximately 2,000 kCals, you do not want to begin a training session or fight with low glycogen stores. You will fatigue early and to a greater extent, and have trouble thinking clearly.

It would be untrue to state that you cannot lose weight through a low-carbohydrate diet, but the weight that is lost is not entirely due to decreased lipid stores and instead will be a result of a combination of significant lean tissue loss, water loss, and lipid loss. Loss of muscle mass will have a strong negative impact on sport performance. There is also no need to take in excess carbohydrates, as excess carbohydrates will be converted to and stored as lipids.

Another commonly used fad diet for weight management is the use of diet pills. Diet pills are considered a supplement and thus fall outside of Food and Drug Administration (FDA) regulations on foods. This allows companies to make blatantly false claims without fear of prosecution. The combination of no FDA oversight and people being desperate to lose weight has resulted in the development of a multibillion-dollar diet pill industry. Over-the-counter diet pills do not work as advertised and can lead to health complications.

It is not recommended to use diet pills as a source of weight management. Not all, but most, diet pills contain stimulants that increase metabolism, which in turn greatly increases resting heart rate and can cause heart palpitations and other medical complications. Because exercise naturally increases heart rate, diet pills can exasperate the increase. On hot, humid days when blood plasma volume drops significantly due to sweating, the use of diet pills can apply excess strain on the heart.

It would be impractical to list and discuss all of the fad diets that are currently being pushed. Thus, I will just give you basic advice that will cover all of them. The first is that if it sounds too good to be true, it most likely is. Weight loss requires time and effort, and there is no substitute. Weight management requires that you increase caloric expenditure through physical activity and eat a well-balanced diet that meets your nutritional needs. Another key concept is that you cannot "target" fat. Fat is fat, and there is no "special" type of fat in the body. You cannot "target" specific storage locations either. There is not a special exercise or diet that will target belly or hip fat. With increases in physical activity you will see an increase in fat stored in muscle, needed for increased energy availability during exercise, and a decrease in adipose storage; however, you cannot target a specific area.

ERGOGENIC AIDS

The word *ergogenic* means work-enhancing. In the arena of sport performance, ergogenic aids are any aid that increases performance. Ergogenic aids affect performance in three basic ways. First, they directly increase performance during an event. Second, they promote recovery between bouts. Lastly, they allow for better training to improve later performance. When considering ergogenic aids, it is important to examine their effectiveness, known and possible side effects, ethics, and legality.

Ethics, Legality, Regulations

Athletes are always focused on finding ways to improve performance, and ergogenic aids provide a pathway for improved performance. Nonetheless, when choosing ergogenic aids the legality and ethics of specific ergogenic aids must be considered. Ethics can be very subjective and are typically based on individual morals and sense of right and wrong. What one person may see as ethical, others may not; however, there is no such gray area when looking at rules and laws. Every sport has a set of rules that competitors must adhere to for them to compete. The United States Anti-Doping Agency (USADA) has a list of banned substances it tests for, discussed in greater detail later in this chapter. There are also laws that prohibit certain substances, for example, steroids.

In sports there is a basic premise that all competition is conducted on an even playing field and that there are no unfair advantages. Any differences in performance should be based strictly on genetics, training, tactics, and ergogenic aids permitted by the sport's governing body. If an ergogenic aid is illegal, for instance, steroids, it is also against regulations and hopefully runs counter to the established ethical guidelines of the athlete.

Most every fight organization in the United States has signed on to the USADA, which is under the World Anti-Doping Agency (WADA). The International Olympic Committee created WADA to regulate the use of ergogenic aids in sports. The charge of this committee is to develop a list of banned substances, set rules, test for banned substances, and enforce rules. The USADA is part of WADA and is responsible for implementing WADA regulations in the United States.

When determining if a substance should be banned, WADA examines three main areas during deliberation:

1. Is the substance illegal?
2. Does the substance pose a serious health risk?

3. Does the substance give the athlete an unfair advantage over their competitors?

An answer of "yes" to one or more of these questions can result in the substance being placed on the banned substance list.

Ultimately, you are responsible for knowing what is on the banned substance list and ensuring that you are not taking a supplement or medication that contains any of the banned substances. The USADA keeps an updated list on what is currently banned in the United States. If you have to take a medication that contains a banned substance, you can file for a therapeutic use exemption.

Supplements

The Dietary Supplement Health and Education Act of 1994 (DSHEA) defined supplements as nonfood, nonfood additive, and nondrug so that they would not fall under the same stringent restrictions as foods. While the FDA has the ability to remove products that have been shown to cause health issues, there are no strict guidelines for production, quality, and content. This act also allows supplement companies to make claims without scientific proof and be intentionally vague. As long as supplement companies do not claim to cure or mitigate a disease, they can make any unsubstantiated claim they desire. DSHEA allows supplements to remain outside of good manufacturing practices (GMP), which requires that all drugs be within a strict limit (typically 1 to 2 percent) of what is stated on the label. Because supplements are not regulated by the FDA for content, many products do not contain the exact volume of specific ingredients as stated on the product label. Scientific studies have examined supplements and found that some have exactly what is stated on the package, while others have little to none of the advertised product.

Due to the way supplements are marketed, it can be difficult to determine what works and what does not. This creates a complicated situation where it is difficult to determine if a specific product will work as advertised, and it is important to look to other sources for information. One common source of information many individuals turn to are the testimonies of professional athletes. Oftentimes professional athletes are paid by the supplement companies to advertise their products. The athlete may or may not actually use the product in their training. The athlete may even believe that the supplement works when it truly has no effect on performance.

Magazines are also not a valid source for information on the effects of ergogenic aids. The magazine may be reluctant to print an article that a supplement does not work when that company is advertising it in its pages. It is not uncommon to see a supplement advertisement written to appear as an article, and in tiny print somewhere on the page you will find something that states it is a paid advertisement.

Peer-reviewed scientific journal articles are the best source of information because the reviewed studies are conducted in strictly controlled settings and an unbiased manner. This can be difficult at times due to not having free access to every journal, and they are often written in such a way that you need a strong understanding of chemistry to be able to understand the article. Textbooks are often a good source, as they have condensed information from various scientific articles into an understandable review of the ergogenic aid.

When looking at scientific articles on the effectiveness of a specific ergogenic aid, make sure to look at multiple studies, as it is common to have varying outcomes. If possible, find a recent review article, as it will have completed all the work for you by examining and comparing the research conducted on that topic.

If you decide to try a specific ergogenic aid, make sure you know the possible side effects, and pay attention to how your body reacts to the supplement. As most supplements are expensive, it would not be cost effective to purchase and use a supplement that has little to no benefit. You will need to calculate a cost–benefit ratio for yourself.

There are a few ergogenic aids that can be beneficial for improving fight performance. A few of those ergogenic aids are mentioned at the beginning of the chapter (water, carbohydrates, proteins, and sports drinks). If you do not think water is an ergogenic aid, try training on a hot day without it and see what happens to your performance. (Joking, don't do that.) Protein is also a vital ergogenic aid, as it greatly assists in anabolic process in the body, aiding in recovery. Carbohydrate ingestion during endurance training has been shown to improve performance during sustained endurance events and is vital for refueling during recovery. Electrolyte replacement is also vital during long events and afterward for recovery.

One ergogenic aid I have not discussed is caffeine. Caffeine is the most widely used supplement in the world. It is a naturally occurring stimulant found in plants (coffee beans, tea leaves, cocoa nuts, etc.). Caffeine is found naturally in many products, including coffee, tea, and soda, but it is often added to other products as a stimulant. Research strongly supports the use of caffeine for improving human performance during endurance sports.

Caffeine can improve performance in three basic ways. The first is that caffeine can easily cross the blood/brain barrier, acting as an ergogenic aid by decreasing feelings of pain and fatigue during exercise, resulting in the ability to compete or train at a higher intensity level. The second is that caffeine both stimulates and increases the mobilization of free fatty acids into the blood, resulting in an increased availability for energy production, conserving glycogen stores. Caffeine increases the ability of the muscles to contract by also increasing activity at the neuromuscular junction and increasing motor unit recruitment.

While caffeine is widely used by a large portion of the population, there are potential side effects. The most common include muscle tremors, gastrointestinal distress, headache, nervousness, elevated heart rate, arrhythmia, and high blood pressure. Side effects are more likely to develop at high levels of ingestion and in individuals who do not normally consume caffeine. While it is commonly stated that caffeine acts as a diuretic, research has shown that caffeine does not act as a diuretic during exercise. This is primarily due to the release of antidiuretic hormone and aldosterone, which occurs during exercise to retain water. The risk of dehydration and thermoregulatory complications are more likely to occur when caffeine ingestion occurs in a hot environment.

It is important to know how your body reacts to caffeine prior to using it as an ergogenic aid, and it should never be used in high dosages. Caffeine does not have to be taken in large doses to increase endurance performance. Caffeine ingestion equivalent to 2.5 cups of coffee has been found to be sufficient to improve performance. Caffeine peaks in the system about one hour after ingestion and therefore should be taken an hour prior to competition. Also be aware that some organizations consider caffeine to be a banned substance. The NCAA has banned caffeine use equivalent to about six to nine 8-ounce cups of coffee. The number of cups will vary depending on the athlete's body mass and timing of ingestion. Do not take caffeine pills, as the quantity of caffeine in a pill is suspect. Anecdotally, I have worked with athletes who were habitual coffee drinkers and experienced negative health consequences when using caffeine pills as an ergogenic aid.

Habitual use of caffeine diminishes the ergogenic effect of it. For those who ingest caffeine (coffee, soda, etc.) on a regular basis, it is recommended to cease caffeine ingestion seven days prior to competition to optimize the effects of caffeine for sports performance.

Illegal Aids

Two illegal ergogenic aids commonly used to improve performance in MMA are anabolic steroids and human growth hormone. This section discusses both ergogenic aids to provide a better understanding of how they work and why you should avoid their use. It is also important to educate yourself on these topics, as they are often discussed in relation to training and competing in elite-level sports.

Anabolic Steroids

Anabolic steroids (synthetic testosterone) are prevalent in all sports—and unfortunately so. Steroids promote anabolic process in the body and improve performance by increasing the speed of recovery, repairing damaged tissue, facilitating greater hypertrophy, and reducing the catabolic effects of exercise. The ability to recover faster between training bouts allows an athlete to train harder more often, which in turn leads to improved performance. Steroids are typically administered through injection, oral doses, patches, or cream.

There are reversible and irreversible side effects that occur with steroid use. Reversible side effects include acne, depression, increased rage, infections at injection sites, and high cholesterol. These side effects dissipate once steroid use has stopped.

The irreversible side effects of steroids occur due to prolonged and heavy use, and are typically more serious. They include cancer, liver disease, cardiovascular disease, and baldness. Side effects that are specific to males are testicular atrophy, impotence, developing mammary glands (breasts), and a permanent decrease in natural testosterone production. Women run the risk of developing facial hair and a deeper voice. Steroid use in pregnant women can also lead to birth defects. Due to the lack of strong scientific research studies in humans, it is not possible to truly know the negative impact steroid use has on health.

Human Growth Hormone

Human growth hormone (HGH) is naturally produced in the body and released from the anterior pituitary. HGH provides two main functions. The first involves anabolic process resulting in tissue growth (muscle, bone, organs). It is believed that the main anabolic effect of HGH is through the stimulation of insulin-like growth factor-1 (IGF-1), which is a major anabolic agent. The second primary function involves metabolism. HGH stimulates lipolysis, reducing the use of glycogen. The combination of these two effects ultimately decreases fat mass while increasing lean body tissue. During exercise, HGH levels naturally increase.

Synthetic HGH was designed to increase growth in individuals experiencing stunted growth response and has since bled into sports performance. Medical use of HGH for increasing growth has demonstrated great promise, with minimal side effects; however, use for sport performance requires a greater volume of HGH, resulting in a significant risk of negative side effects. Common side effects found with the use of synthetic HGH are enlarged heart, enlarged bone structures, arthritis, insulin resistance, and carpal tunnel syndrome.

6

COMPETITION

This chapter covers areas of basic knowledge when it comes to choosing fights and preparing for competition. There is a lot more to preparing for a competition than one might think. You must find a fight, get a license for that state, obtain medical clearance, arrange the logistics, and make weight. This chapter provides a basic outline to give a generalized idea of what is needed logistically. You will need to work with your coach to make sure that the details are properly addressed for your upcoming fight. Fighting strategies are beyond the scope of this book and not discussed in this chapter. It is important that you work with your coach to develop a fight strategy that focuses on your strengths and acknowledges your opponent's strengths and weaknesses.

CHOOSING A FIGHT

If you are new to mixed martial arts (MMA) you can expect one to two years of training prior to your first fight. It is important that you gain adequate skill sets, tactical knowledge, and fitness level prior to your first fight. Fighting too soon can damage a fighter both physically and psychologically. Fighters who are not adequately prepared for a fight will experience more physical damage in relation to a fighter who is adequately prepared to fight. Experiencing a really bad fight your first time out can negatively impact your confidence, making it more difficult to fight again. Listen to your coach, as he will be able to make an educated and unbiased decision about your preparedness to fight. Win or lose, you want to walk into the fight optimally prepared and not overwhelmingly outmatched.

Once you and your coach determine that you are ready for your first fight, you must determine the opponent you wish to fight or the tournament you wish to compete in. For starting amateurs, it is not realistic to believe that you will be able to choose your opponent for every fight; however, do not agree to a fight in which you are grievously overmatched. It will be more beneficial to your fighting career to decline a fight when you are knowingly outmatched. Be patient and wait for a fight with an opponent who is a good match.

Unless you live in an area with a large MMA scene, you will need to be willing to travel to find fights that will allow you to grow as a fighter. In areas where there is not a large MMA scene, there will be few opportunities to fight, and the opportunities you do get may not be good ones. In smaller areas, the better you become as a fighter, the fewer fights you will be able to find locally, as you will find fewer opponents willing to fight you. Too often fighters limit themselves to their local area and will not travel to grow their skill set and improve their record.

When possible, choose fights that are officially sanctioned by the athletic committee of that state, since they will follow Association of Boxing Commissions regulations. In general, sanctioned fights will be better organized and safer for all fighters involved. This will ensure that all fighters are healthy and ready to fight, and that the fight will follow the Unified Rules of Mixed Martial Arts.

LOGISTICS

There are various logistical concerns you will need to address when preparing for a fight. Some of the more basic logistical considerations are simple but time consuming. Until you become a professional fighter with a dedicated manager, all the work is your responsibility. You will need to make travel and lodging arrangements for yourself and your corner team. Choose lodging that provides easy access to the fight venue, as well as any other local accommodations you require. You will need to know the registration requirements, deadline, and fees, and address those accordingly.

Spend time researching the fight and the organization. It is important that you know the rules and regulations for the organization in which you are fighting. Most all sanctioned fights will follow the Unified Rules of Mixed Martial Arts; however, different organizations have differing rule sets. For example, One Championship allows knees to a grounded opponent's head, whereas Ultimate Fighting Championship does not. Bellator follows the Unified Rules of Mixed Martial Arts, but they do not allow elbows to the head during the early stages of the tournament, as a cut fighter could not advance in the tournament. You do not want to be disqualified because you are unaware of the rule set specific to your fight.

Prefight Requirements

Aside from registration and associated fees, there are other prefight requirements you should be aware of. These requirements will vary by state and organization, and are often time consuming. Because requirements do vary, it is important that you do your research and determine what you need to accomplish prior to your fight. Some of the more common requirements are as follows:

- *Required licensing through the state athletic commission.* Each state has their own athletic commission, and you will need to obtain a license for the state in which you are planning to fight. The organization hosting your fight should be able to supply the information you need. If the organization does not provide the information, you can contact the athletic commission directly.
- *Physical exam and medical clearance.* It is important that all fighters report to the fight healthy; therefore, physical exams and medical clearance are required. Medical screening not only makes sure you are physically able to fight safely, but also eliminates fighters who have easily transmittable blood-borne pathogens. Oftentimes regulations will require that older fighters obtain more in-depth testing to ensure they are ready to fight. Some of the most common tests required are the following:
  - Basic physical
  - Blood work
  - Neurological exam
  - Eye exam
  - Pregnancy test
- *Proof of skill level.* Many organizations will require proof of skill level to permit you to fight. The most common acceptable methods of proving skill level are a fight record, fight footage, or a signed letter from an acceptable source stating your skill level (e.g., your coach).

Making Weight

To keep fights both fair and safe, weight classes were developed. Weight classes allow for the pairing of similar-sized individuals to prevent one fighter from being overpowered by another. This allows the fight to be determined more by physical attributes, skill level, and strategy than size differentials. The typical male weight classes you will find in MMA are as follows:

flyweight (115–125 pounds)
bantamweight (125–135 pounds)
featherweight (135–145 pounds)
lightweight (145–155 pounds)
welterweight (155–170 pounds)
middleweight (170–185 pounds)
light heavyweight (185–205 pounds)
heavyweight (205–265 pounds)
super heavyweight (≥265 pounds)

The typical female weight classes you will find in MMA are the following:

atomweight (≤105 pounds)
strawweight (105–115 pounds)
flyweight (115–125 pounds)
bantamweight (125–135 pounds)
featherweight (135–145 pounds)

Once weight classes were established it did not take fighters long to understand that you want more muscle mass and less fat within any given weight class. It is the lean body mass that really matters when you are looking at opponents in any given weight class. As stated previously, lean body mass consists of all components of the body minus fat (muscle, bone, organs, etc.). There is a large difference between a fighter who is 180 pounds at 4 percent body fat and a second fighter who is 180 pounds at 18 percent body fat. When looking at lean body mass, the first fighter would have 172.8 pounds of lean body mass, and the second fighter would have 147.6 pounds of lean body mass. If the fighters are of similar height, the vast majority of the 25.2-pound difference is muscle. From this example you can easily see the advantage of being as lean as possible in any given weight class.

You and your coach will determine what weight class best suites your individual body. The ideal is to choose a weight class that does not require a large weight cut yet gives you a physical advantage over your opponent. When determining weight class, you will need to take into account your current weight and your desired weight. Pick a realistic weight class that allows you to easily stay within that class.

Weight cutting is used to drop weight to make weight prior to your fight. Once you accept a fight in a specific weight class, you must present yourself to weigh in for that specific weight class. If you miss weight, you can be disqualified or fined. If it is a title fight and you miss weight and are allowed to fight, you will be fined and be ineligible to compete for the title. In many cases, it is up to your opponent to allow the fight to happen or not if you miss weight. These facts put a heavy burden on the fighter to make weight on fight night. This is also why it is important to fight in a weight class where drastic weight cuts are not necessary to make weight.

Before I discuss methods of weight cutting, it is important to talk about the negative consequences of weight cutting. Severe weight cutting can be dangerous, resulting in fatigue, illness, impaired cognitive function, overall decrease in performance, and possible death. No one can significantly cut to make weight and perform at their peak level, as full physical recovery from severe weight cutting is not possible prior to a fight. The risks are serious enough that One Championship chose to regulate weight cutting by monitoring their athletes' weight and hydration levels, and requiring that their fighters fight at their normal walk-around weight. Severe weight cutting will disqualify one of their fighters from fighting. Due to the dangers and significant decreases in performance that occur from severe weight cuts it is important to fight in a weight class that is as close as possible to your walk-around weight. To accomplish that goal, it becomes important to maintain a healthy fight weight throughout the year, avoiding massive fluctuations in weight.

In the following sections I discuss both long-term weight loss and weight cutting. There are distinct differences between the two. Long-term weight loss is done through exercise and manipulation of caloric intake during an extended period of time. Weight cutting is conducted immediately prior to weigh-in where you manipulate hydration levels to lose weight and then rehydrate right after weigh-in. If possible, I recommend working with a sport nutritionist to optimize weight loss while optimizing performance gains and remaining healthy. Prior to making any drastic changes in diet it is important to consult your physician. This statement is especially true if you have any known medical conditions that could be affected by drastic changes in diet.

Long-Term Weight Loss

Long-term weight loss is considered any weight loss that occurs throughout time as opposed to immediately prior to weigh-in. This will be a meaningful loss of body fat as opposed to short-term water loss. The length of time for long-term weight loss could be anywhere from a month to multiple years and will be highly dependent on the individual and the individual's goals. The details of weight management are discussed in chapter 5, "Nutrition for Mixed Martial Arts."

The first step is to evaluate where you are currently. Look at both your weight and body fat percentage. These numbers will allow you to make an educated decision about your desired weight class and the path you will need to take to reach that goal. For example, let's look at a beginning fighter who weighs 180 pounds at 18 percent body fat and wants to fight at welterweight. He sets his long-term goal to drop his weight from 180 pounds to 160 pounds and his body fat from 18 percent to 7 percent. Attempting to drop 20 pounds in a short period of time would be too much. Instead, set a long-term goal for the span of a year and work on keeping the fighter on track. It is okay if the fighter reaches his goal in less than a year. The key is to slowly progress in a healthy manner. Also, keep in mind that with a year of proper training, the fighter will put on more muscle; therefore, their lean body weight will increase. They may end up at 165 pounds at 7 percent body fat as opposed to the original goal of 160 pounds and 7 percent body fat. For this reason, it is important to monitor changes in not only weight, but also body fat, as it will also give you information on changes in lean body mass. For this process to work it is important that you have a valid and reliable scale. A scale can be reliable (meaning that you can step on and off the scale and each time you get the same number) yet not valid (meaning that it indicates you are 180 pounds when in actuality you are 190 pounds). Make sure your scale is calibrated and accurate.

You can also plan a long-term weight cut for a shorter period of time after you establish your walk-around weight. For this example I will use a welterweight fighter (155–170 pounds) whose walk-around weight is 178 pounds at 10 percent body fat. The goal would be to drop 8 to 10 pounds during the span of the 2 months leading up to the fight through altered diet and the increase in training volume and intensity that would naturally occur leading up to a fight. Getting the fighter down to 168 to 170 pounds at 4 to 6 percent body fat will get him where he needs to be without a drastic weight cut for the official weigh-in. Try not to cut too much too quickly, as it will negatively impact both training and training adaptations. Also monitor the quality and timing of nutrition during this time period.

Determining your walk-around weight and weight class is extremely important because you do not want to have to make drastic weight cuts to make weigh-in. If you weigh 185 at 4 percent body fat it is unrealistic that you can easily drop 15 pounds during a weight cut to fight welterweight, as that is an 8.1 percent water cut. If you do make the cut, chances are strong that you will not fight near your full capacity. I would advise fighting at middleweight, putting on 5 more pounds of muscle (it will take time), and then cutting to 185 pounds for weigh-in.

Weight Cut

Weight cutting differs from long-term weight loss in that takes place in a much shorter period of time and focuses on reduced water content in the body to make weight at the official weigh-in. The idea of weight cutting is that you will shed water to make the desired weight class, rehydrate, and then fight at a much heavier weight. As the weigh-in typically occurs the day prior to the fight, it gives the fighter approximately 24 hours to rehydrate; however, this is not enough time to fully recover physically from drastic weight cuts. When weigh-in is the same day as the fight, adequate rehydration is impossible. Oftentimes professional fighters will use intravenous solution to rehydrate, as ingesting fluids alone is not sufficient to rehydrate by fight time.

As stated earlier in this book, a decrease in water equivalent to 2 percent of body mass will negatively impact performance, and a decrease to 5 percent will negatively impact health. If you have a fighter that weighs 179 pounds, they will need to drop 9 pounds to make weight for a welterweight fight, which is 5 percent of their body mass. It is not uncommon for professional fighters to exceed a 5 percent weight cut within a 24-hour period to make weight, resulting in health risk and poor performance. Any combat athlete who has had to drop a drastic amount of weight will tell you that it was worse on them than the training leading up to the fight and the fight itself.

Before I talk about weight cutting, I would like to state that I strongly advise against using drastic weight cuts to make weight, as it puts you at risk for health issues and will decrease your performance during the fight. It is simply not worth the risk. There are numerous methods for cutting water weight prior to weigh-in. In the past the most commonly used methods were to sit in a sauna and sweat profusely or work out in a sweat suit that allowed little to no evaporation to occur, resulting in heavy water loss, or a combination of the two methods. These methods are not advisable given that they put too much strain on the system and recovery from these methods prior to a fight is almost impossible. In recent history, water loading has become the preferred method for weight cutting, as it produces results and is safer in relation to exercising in a sauna while wearing a sweat suit.

Water loading is the process of greatly increasing water intake for three to five days prior to weigh-in and then ceasing water intake, with the result being a decrease in body mass. This system uses the body's response to hydration levels to assist in water loss. The body maintains homeostasis (an internal autoregulation process to maintain balance throughout the body) and does not like to deviate from a set norm. There is a specific temperature, pH, blood glucose level, hydration, electrolyte level, and so on, that the body must maintain for normal function. The act of water loading takes the body out of homeostasis by causing abnormally high hydration levels due to excess water intake.

One of the main hormones that adjusts to excess water intake is vasopressin (an antidiuretic hormone), which cause greater water retention in the kidneys. During exercise in the heat, vasopressin is activated to retain water by decreased urination to assist in the prevention of dehydration; however, during water loading the release of vasopressin from the neurohypophysis is greatly inhibited due to high water concentrations in the body. High water concentrations will dilute sodium concentrations, resulting in an electrolyte imbalance, which is undesirable. A reduction in vasopressin release will result in a significant increase in urination so that water can be excreted quickly to maintain homeostasis.

As stated earlier, the process requires that water intake increases three to five days prior to weigh-in. The recommendation of three to five days will be based on how much you need to cut and how your body responds to water loading. It is recommended that you drink about 100 ml of water per kg of body mass each day during the loading period. For example, if you have a 180-pound individual who needs to cut weight for an upcoming fight, you would use the following calculations:

180 pounds ÷ 2.205 = 81.63 kg
81.63 kg × 100 = 8,163.3 ml or 8.16 L

The next step in the process occurs prior to weigh-in. The day prior to weigh-in, restrict water intake to about 10 to 20 ml/kg of body mass. Use the aforementioned formula to calculate water intake for the day. In the example with the 180-pound fighter, the water intake would be between .82 L and 1.63 L. The body will still be responding to lower vasopressin, and urination will still be high, resulting in water loss and therefore weight loss. The following morning you will cease water intake until weigh-in and then immediately begin rehydrating. If you are not weighing in until late at night, you may want to ingest water earlier that morning and cease water consumption later in the day. It is important to note that if your weigh-in time is right before competition, water loading will not work, as you will not have time to replenish prior to competition.

While water loading relies on predictable physiological responses, it not an exact science when it comes to precise volume of water lost. It is important that you understand how your body responds to the water-loading method prior to your first fight. Do a trial run well before your first fight so you know about how much water weight you will drop and how our body responds to loading, unloading, and refueling.

While fighters typically respond better to water loading as opposed to other methods, there are still risks involved. There is always a risk when you manipulate hormones in the body. It is important to be careful during the water-loading period and not ingest too much water, as a consequence could be hyponatremia (low sodium in relation to water). When hyponatremia is present, high fluid levels dilute sodium levels, resulting in the swelling of cells. Hyponatremia can result in serious illness and death. If hyponatremia is suspected, seek medical attention immediately. The following are symptoms of hyponatremia:

- Headache
- Nausea
- Cramping
- Seizures
- Coma

Along with water loading, you can also lower carbohydrates for the week leading up to weigh-in. As mentioned in chapter 5, carbohydrates are essential for training and performance, and you should stay away from low- and no-carbohydrate diets. This fact still holds true, but you will not need as many carbohydrates during the week leading up to the fight, as you will be tapering with lower intensity and volume. You will need to make sure to replenish carbohydrate stores after weigh-in prior to the fight. I recommend only cutting carbohydrates in the week leading up to weigh-in if weigh-in occurs the day prior to the fight. You must have adequate time to replenish your diminished stores prior to competition.

WARMING UP FOR A FIGHT

It is vitally important that you warm up prior to your fight and keep your heart rate up prior to the bell. The benefits of a warm-up are discussed earlier in this book, but I will quickly touch on the importance again here. The primary reasons to warm up are to increase heart rate, blood flow to the working muscles, and heat generated within the muscles. These mechanisms are designed to prepare the body for work. You need at least two minutes to steady state, but you will spend more time than that warming up.

Spend 5 to 10 minutes with an easy cardio warm-up like jogging or jumping rope, keeping intensity very low. Next you will want to perform dynamic stretching covering the entire body for about 5 minutes. Upon completion of your dynamic stretching, spend about 10 minutes going through skill drills to finish off your warm-up. You want to time your warm-up so that you finish when it is time to head to the ring. Do not allow a long time period to pass with inactivity prior to the start of the fight, as it will negate your warm-up.

PSYCHOLOGICAL READINESS

It is normal to experience nervousness and anxiety prior to a fight. This feeling occurs in all sports prior to competition; however, there are no other sports that are as raw as combat sports. MMA requires that you demonstrate your tactical fighting skills, combat tactical knowledge, and ability to take damage in a scenario where it is just you and your opponent in front of everyone. It is not a team sport where your mistakes can be hidden among the other players, and you are the sole recipient of the consequences of those mistakes. Oftentimes fighters are more afraid of looking bad in the eyes of spectators than being injured. That does not mean fighters are not afraid of being injured; every fighter knows that injury is part of the sport.

These fears will exist prior to every fight. The trick is to accept the possibility of loss and injury, and not dwell on those thoughts. Instead, spend the time focusing on your skill sets and warming up. Treat it as you would any warm-up, and do not overthink the outcome of the fight, as it is impossible to determine the verdict ahead of time. Focus on what you already know; there is no new skill or tactic you can learn right before the fight that would be beneficial.

This will sound counterproductive at first, as well as almost impossible to accomplish, but you must learn to relax during the warm-up and stay relaxed throughout the fight. The more tense you are, the slower your movements will become. While a tensed muscle can produce force, it decreases speed, resulting in reduced power and more predictable movements. There are many different relaxation techniques you can implement, for instance, visualization and breathing techniques. You will need to find one that works well for you.

Stay away from negative thoughts; they are self-defeating and a distraction from your goal. Shut down all negative thoughts, as they are not beneficial to your fight, and focus on the positive. Moreover, do not spend a lot of time with inspirational talks. Too long an inspirational talk from your coach or too much internal inspirational self-talk can be distracting and remove your focus from where it needs to be. A short "you got this" talk or positive thought is fine, but do not drone on. It is much more productive to go through tactical and technical training. Focusing on possible positive or negative outcomes of a fight is not productive. Your time will be better spent focusing on physically warming up and working through your technical and tactical skills.

7

SPECIAL CONSIDERATIONS FOR TRAINING AND COMPETITION

In previous chapters I discuss how the body responds and adapts to exercise. This information applies to everyone in general, but it may need to be modified based on such factors as, age, gender, disease state, or disability. This chapter covers special considerations for specific populations that require adaptation to their training program to be successful. Due to gender differences, males and females respond slightly different to training. As we age, the body is altered and will not adapt to training in the same manner; therefore, training programs must adapt. Specific disease states alter the body's ability to adapt and may require special care and consideration. Certain biomechanical and physiological adaptations must be made when working with disabled athletes as well.

WOMEN

Female participation in sports has increased dramatically. Mixed martial arts (MMA) is one sport where female participation has grown exponentially. When developing a training program for females, the same training principles discussed earlier can be applied without alterations. Women adapt to training stimuli in ways that are very similar to male athletes; however, there are distinct differences and a few key factors that should be taken into consideration when developing a training program.

Differences in Sex

We should begin by acknowledging that there are key physiological differences between males and females. One of the primary differences between males and females involves hormones, primarily testosterone and estrogen. Males naturally produce 10 times more testosterone than females. Greater volumes of testosterone result in greater anabolic processes and therefore a significantly larger increase in muscle mass. Men can produce a faster contraction than females due to a greater speed of signaling, resulting in greater power. As power increases, so does the effectiveness of strikes. Distribution of muscle mass also differs between males and females. A greater percentage of muscle mass is distributed in the upper body in males. It is important to note that there are no physiological differences between male and female muscle tissue, and the main difference in muscle mass is directly related to hormone levels. When looking at absolute strength, men are, on average, 30 to 60 percent stronger than females. These numbers are based on the average population. When looking at peer groups (fighters of the same level and weight), the percentage differences are on the lower end; however, when you make the comparison based on weight lifted in relation to lean body mass, the differences diminish significantly.

Oftentimes women are concerned with becoming "bulky" or "looking like a guy" from resistance training. Thus, they will avoid any form of resistance training. This is an unfounded concern, as women do not produce anywhere near the same volume of testosterone that males do and therefore will not "bulk up" with resistance training designed for MMA. A female would have to develop a resistance training program specifically designed for bulking up to achieve that goal. Due to hormonal differences, it is much more difficult for females to put on muscle mass.

While females do not produce large amounts of testosterone, they do produce a large volume of estrogen, which affects the way females develop physiologically. One of the key roles of estrogen is increased lipid storage, particularly in the thighs and hips. This is the reason that essential body fat in females is 12 percent as opposed to 4 percent in males. Increased lipid storage is essential for the reproductive process. This is also why you can have a female fighter and male fighter of the same weight but the male fighter is stronger, because a greater percentage of his weight will be lean muscle mass. Keep in mind that this statement is assuming that both fighters are of the same level and at their fight weight. Estrogen also plays an important part in female bone growth, increasing calcium storage and retention.

Females have a lower aerobic capacity in relation to their male counterparts. There are several factors that attribute to this phenomenon. The first is that males possess a larger overall blood volume and increased hemoglobin count per milliliter of blood in relation to females. A greater hemoglobin count increases oxygen-carrying capacity, which in turn increases performance. To help offset lower levels of hemoglobin, females typically have higher levels of 2,3-DPG, which helps release oxygen into the tissue more easily. Nonetheless, this does not completely compensate for the gender difference. Women also tend to have smaller hearts, which in turn decreases stroke volume. These factors lead to a lower aerobic capacity, resulting in lower VO_2 max measures. At any given fitness level, females will produce VO_2 max scores that will be 5 to 10 ml/kg/min lower than their male counterparts.

While sex differences are scientifically verified, it does not mean that all males can outperform all females. The key is that males possess a higher aerobic capacity, greater lean muscle mass, and faster activation at any given level of competition. It is possible for a pro female fighter to defeat an amateur-level male fighter in the same weight class; however, a female professional fighter would have difficulty with a pro male fighter of the same level. This is why there are male and female divisions. Moreover, keep in mind that while physical performance is very important in MMA, skill is king.

Female Athlete Triad

One of the common concerns for female athletes is the female athlete triad. As the name suggests, the triad consist of three distinct but interlocking components: inadequate caloric intake, amenorrhea, and osteoporosis. The process begins with inadequate caloric intake. Athletes expend a lot of calories, and when caloric expenditure consistently and excessively exceeds caloric intake, it creates a negative balance, resulting in an unhealthy body composition. As mentioned earlier, 12 percent body fat is considered essential in females. Those who drop below this percentage run the risk of developing the female athlete triad, as well as other health discrepancies. This caloric imbalance is commonly brought on by the desire to optimize performance, as well as concerns with body image.

The desire to optimize body composition for performance and body image can become an obsession and lead to eating disorders like anorexia nervosa and bulimia. More than half of female athletes have been diagnosed with eating disorders; however, you do not have to have an eating disorder to be in a constant negative caloric balance. Training for MMA has a high caloric cost and therefore requires a high caloric intake. A female fighter may appear to eat normally but still be in a negative caloric balance. When eating disorders are present, there is a strong psychological aversion to food or what food represents to that individual. In this case, the psychological aversion does not exist; they are just not eating adequately. Weight cutting leading up to a fight will put a female at risk for the development of the female athlete triad. It is a good idea to monitor caloric expenditure, as well as caloric intake. Another way is to monitor body composition to ensure that you maintain essential body fat.

The next component of the female athlete triad is the development of abnormalities in the menstrual cycle, ultimately leading to amenorrhea (cessation of the menstrual cycle). Prolonged negative caloric balance and unhealthy body composition has a negative impact on the hypothalamus, reducing the release of gonadotropic hormones, which in turn impacts estrogen production and the menstrual cycle. An unhealthy body composition does not have to exist for amenorrhea to occur. A high training volume or high-intensity training has also been shown to lead to amenorrhea.

The final component of the female athlete triad is the development of osteoporosis, where bone density decreases, causing bone to become brittle and easily fractured. Estrogen is responsible for the absorption and retention of calcium. When estrogen production greatly decreases with the cessation of the menstrual cycle, calcium absorption and retention greatly diminish, leading to a decrease in bone density. While the female athlete triad is a serious concern for females of all ages, special attention should be paid to those in their developmental years, when bone growth is paramount.

Female Biomechanics

One of the main structural differences between males and females is the pelvic girdle. Women have a wider pelvic girdle and sacrum, and the pelvis is shaped slightly differently. These differences are necessary to accommodate the birth process. These factors also lead to altered lower extremity biomechanics and greater risk of lower extremity injuries in relation to males. Knee injuries (primarily anterior cruciate ligament [ACL] ruptures) are more prevalent in female athletes. Female athletes are six to eight times more likely to rupture an ACL than male athletes of the same sport. This is especially true in MMA. One method for decreasing the risk of injury is to strengthen the knee extensors (quadriceps) and knee flexors (hamstrings). Typically, the quadriceps muscles are significantly stronger than the hamstring muscles. Research supports that the less the strength difference between the extensors and flexors the less likely it is that an injury will occur.

Pregnancy

Research has demonstrated that there are many benefits for women who exercise during pregnancy. Some of the proposed benefits are a decrease in excessive weight gain, decreased labor pains, decreased risk of developing gestational diabetes, and easier return to prepregnancy weight and fitness level after birth. Exercise during pregnancy should only be conducted by females who are experiencing a normal pregnancy and have their doctor's permission. Remember, only your doctor can determine if you are healthy enough to exercise and at what level you can train.

Once you become pregnant, sit down and have an honest and detailed conversation with your doctor concerning exercise. Once it has been established that you are experiencing a normal, healthy pregnancy, discuss your goals and training plan with your doctor. The doctor will establish your training limitations, which you should follow precisely. Throughout the pregnancy continue to maintain a continuous and open dialogue regarding your training.

Once you become pregnant, your training goals will need to be altered to accommodate your current state. You will need to eliminate any form of contact or risk of impact from your training. As pregnancy progresses, balance becomes compromised. As the baby grows and the belly protrudes, the body's center of gravity shifts. The hormone relaxin is released to relax the pelvis to prepare for birth. Unfortunately, relaxin also causes other joints in the lower extremities to loosen, which leads to decreased stability and balance.

Your training intensity will also need to be lowered. Blood flow is redirected during exercise to the working muscles and skin for cooling, which in turn reduces blood flow to the fetus. At mild to moderate intensity, reduced blood flow does not impact fetus health; however, as intensity increases, a greater amount of blood is redirected from the uterus. It is for this reason that vigorous, high-intensity exercise should be avoided during pregnancy. When training, it is okay to exercise until you feel slightly fatigued, but never exercise to exhaustion. Due to alterations in blood flow during pregnancy, heart rate becomes an unreliable tool for determining exercise intensity. Instead, use perceived exertion to determine intensity.

Due to reduced blood flow to the skin and increased insulation, your ability to dissipate heat is greatly compromised during pregnancy. A significant increase in the fetus's core temperature can negatively impact development. Do not train in the heat, stay well hydrated, and be mindful of any significant increase in core temperature. Train during a cooler part of the day or inside to avoid overheating.

Exercise in a supine position, on your back, is also not recommended during pregnancy, as it lowers cardiac output and can restrict blood flow to the fetus. Find an alternate exercise to replace those you typically conduct in a supine position.

AGING

Aging has a strong impact on our ability to adapt to training. We are all on a theoretical curve where physical abilities increase through life until they peak somewhere between the ages of 25 and 30 years old. We can briefly maintain that peak until our physical abilities begin to gradually decline between the ages of 35 and 40. This curve remains true for all healthy individuals. Naturally, someone who trains will have a higher performance level at any point in the curve when compared to a sedentary individual.

Fitness level along this curve can be altered by increasing or decreasing physical activity. If a collegiate athlete who has been active his entire life stopped training after college, his fitness level would eventually drop back down to the level of someone who is sedentary. The reverse is true for someone who has been sedentary his entire life and decides to start training. But the basic principle still remains true that your ability to adapt to training will begin to diminish at approximately age 35, with a significant decline starting at about 45 years of age.

Aerobic capacity decreases significantly with age. It is estimated that there is a reduction in VO_2 max of approximately 1 ml/kg/min a year. Much of the age-related decrease in VO_2 max is due to the substantial reduction in physical activity that occurs as an individual ages. Those who remain active throughout life can offset the loss in VO_2 max, which occurs due to a reduction in physical activity. While not as steep a decline, those who remain active will still see a reduction in aerobic capacity due to a reduction in cardiovascular function and an age-related decrease in muscle mass (sarcopenia).

Sarcopenia is a common component of aging; however, the extent of the decline in muscle mass is highly dependent on the individual's fitness level. For those who remain active throughout life, the decrease is lessened. While physical activity goes a long way toward preventing loss of muscle mass, it cannot completely offset sarcopenia. The aging process results in a significant decrease in hormone production, resulting in a decrease in protein synthesis and, thus, a decrease in muscle mass.

With age there is a naturally occurring decrease in bone density. There are two distinct stages: osteopenia and osteoporosis. Osteopenia is a decrease in bone density that occurs prior to the development of osteoporosis and is much less severe. At this stage, bones are more susceptible to damage than normal bone but less susceptible than bones in an osteoporotic state. Osteoporosis is a severe decrease in bone density that causes greater susceptibility to fracture. Both states occur due to age-related decreases in hormones. In males, there is a link between an age-related decrease in testosterone production and a decrease in bone density. In females, there is a strong relationship between estrogen levels and bone density. This leaves postmenopausal women strongly suscep-tible to the development of osteoporosis due to a sizable decrease in estrogen production postmenopause. Estrogen is a key hormone in the absorption and retention of calcium in females. Since estrogen production is greatly dimin-ished, the absorption and retention of calcium decreases, leading to a reduction in bone density.

There are two main areas that you can address to help prevent a decrease in bone density. First, maintain a healthy, well-balanced diet. Second, participate in weight-bearing activities. Bones respond to stress in the basic manner that muscle does. If you apply adequate mechanical stress to the bone, bone den-sity increases. If inadequate mechanical stress is applied to bone, bone density decreases. Weight-bearing activity is the only way to increase bone density. Ex-amples of weight-bearing activities are running, lifting, plyometrics, and heavy bag workouts. Running is a weight-bearing activity that can lead to increased bone density; however, the mechanical stress is focused on the lower body and does nothing to increase bone density in the upper body. Thus, when develop-ing a program with bone density in mind, it is important to choose activities that will apply a mechanical load for the entire body. Resistance training is weight-bearing and allows for adequate stress to be applied to almost every bone in the body. In MMA, training on the heavy bag is another method that will apply an overall mechanical load to the body as punches, elbows, knees, and kicks are employed during the workout.

These recommendations are not guaranteed protection against the develop-ment of osteopenia and osteoporosis. There is also a genetic component for the development of these disorders; however, maintaining a proper diet and includ-ing weight-bearing activities in your training are vital steps toward maintaining proper bone density. Keep in mind that MMA is a contact sport in which it is important to maintain bone density to offset the risk of fractures due to training and competition.

A significant decrease in cardiac output occurs with aging. This decrease is as a result of diminished stroke volume and maximal heart rate. The age-related decrease in stroke volume occurs due to a reduction in the left ventricle's ability to expand and contract, with the result being less blood ejected from the heart during each beat. At the same time, there is an estimated decrease in maximal heart rate by one beat per minute each year. The decrease in maximal heart rate is believed to be attributed to age-related changes to the cardiac conduction system (the electrical signaling for contraction), combined with decreased sensitivity of the myocardium to specific hormones, primarily epinephrine and norepinephrine. A decrease in cardiac output results in a corresponding decrease in aerobic performance.

Another key factor in the age-related decline in performance is ability to recover between training bouts, resulting in a decrease in an individual's ability to handle higher volumes and intensities. Monitor your response to training as you age, and adapt the triaging program accordingly. There will come a point where both intensity and volume will need to be adjusted to allow time for adequate recovery. The exact timing is variable and will be highly dependent on your age, training status, health, and training goals.

There is a decrease in neuromuscular response as you age. In MMA you will notice diminished performance in reaction times, neuromuscular recruitment patterns, and speed of contraction. The greatest impact is seen in voluntary muscle responses to a stimulus. An example would be slipping a jab. As you age, your ability to recognize the jab may not be diminished, but your ability to initiate the proper response quickly and efficiently will be. Staying physically active will offset this decline, but it will not completely negate it.

Flexibility also decreases as we age. There are various reasons flexibility decreases with age, problems at the joints, decrease in elasticity of the muscle, and so forth. The primary reason for a decrease in flexibility as we age is directly related to lack of flexibility training. If you want to stay flexible as you age, you need to stretch as you age.

Do not let age-related decreases in performance discourage you from pursuing your goals. Use this information to help develop a training program that will optimize your increases in performance. Keep in mind that increases in performance can occur at any age and therefore should not hinder anyone from starting a program. It is important to note that fitness gains for someone beginning a training program at 45 will not occur as quickly or be as large as an individual who started a program at 20, assuming both are using the same program. Training can lead to increases in muscle mass, decreases in body fat, increases in bone density, and lower blood pressure, and can positively impact cholesterol levels and provide many other health benefits. While medical clearance is important at every age, it is vitally important that older individuals consult a physician prior to beginning an exercise program.

CHILDREN AND ADOLESCENCE

For the purpose of this chapter, childhood is defined as age six to puberty, and adolescence is defined as the time period from puberty to 18 years of age. Getting our youth involved in physical activity at an early age is extremely important, and MMA is an excellent way to get them involved. All of my boys have been involved in martial arts since an early age. Some continue to train, and others have found other interests. I highly encourage everyone to get their kids involved in martial arts for the physical, psychological, and practical benefits.

I am often asked at what age children should begin martial arts. My answer is always that it depends on your child. The typical age to start martial arts is about six years old, but it is not about biological age. Instead, it has more to do with the child's neuromuscular coordination and ability to follow directions. Neuromuscular coordination improves as the child ages and they have better control of their movements. It is important that the movements the child is attempting to learn are age appropriate so that they do not become frustrated with the activity. The child must also be able to focus enough to learn and not distract other students. Keep in mind that no child will be perfectly behaved, focused, and on task the entire time. The keys are to keep it fun so that they learn, keep them on task as much as possible, and help them understand that mastering martial arts is a long road and there is no need to try to sprint forward.

Children and adolescents differ from adults both physiologically and psychologically. It is important to understand these differences, as children should not be trained as small adults. The main physiological difference involves hormone levels. Prior to puberty, children produce very small amounts of hormones and therefore cannot adapt to training as effectively as adults. Research has demonstrated that performance gains in prepubescent children occur in areas of aerobic performance, anaerobic performance, muscular endurance, and muscular strength; however, the mechanisms behind these improvements occur through physiological pathways that are slightly, but importantly, different than adults.

With endurance training, children can experience significant gains in aerobic performance, but with these gains there is little to no change in their aerobic capacity or VO_2 max measurements. Instead, increases in aerobic performance are attributed to improved neuromuscular recruitment patterns. As the child's technique improves, he becomes more economical, and aerobic performance improves dramatically with no alteration to aerobic capacity.

This same basic concept applies to resistance training as well. With resistance training, children can see an increase in both muscular strength and muscular endurance. This increase in strength is not due to muscle hypertrophy, but instead occurs as a result of neuromuscular adaptations that occur through training. Children younger than age 13 should only be doing muscular endurance resistance training and should not be lifting heavy.

The overall key message is that training for children should not focus on attempting to alter aerobic capacity or strength. Instead, the training programs should focus on producing proper technique, leading to optimizing recruitment patterns.

Training for kids should focus on having fun while learning. At this stage, training should not feel like a chore, and children should look forward to it. The biggest mistake people make is forcing training on children and working them too hard. Watch and listen to your child; he will let you know when he is tired and needs a break.

During puberty, hormone levels begin to increase. As a child reaches adolescence, his ability to adapt to training, beyond just neuromuscular, improves dramatically. During puberty, male testosterone production increases to about 10 times that of prepubescent levels, resulting in a substantially increased rate of growth. During this period, joints may not be as stable, which may result in pain and possible injury during sports. Once puberty is reached, both volume and intensity can increase but not yet to the level of an adult. An adolescent can begin an entry-level adult program at 16 years of age. This is an average age, and programs should be individualized, as some adolescents mature faster or slower than others.

Another aspect to consider when working with youth is that they are still developing psychologically. Children and adolescents may not be able to readily grasp complicated concepts, so keep the explanations simple and expressed in terms they can understand. This will not only get the concept across to them, but also prevent the child from becoming frustrated.

Avoid training intensities and volumes that are too high. Sports-related injuries have drastically increased in children due to improper training volumes. Children are developing overuse injuries that typically do not occur in athletes until their collegiate or professional careers. One of the primary reasons is that adult training programs are being applied to children and adolescents. Another principal reason is that kids are playing sports at a high volume and intensity year-round. It is highly recommended that children stay active year-round, and

MMA is an excellent way to do this; however, it is important to keep track of the overall training volume and intensity to prevent overtraining and overuse injuries. Not every training session needs to be high intensity. It is also important to account for your child's other sports when considering overall training load.

OVERWEIGHT AND OBESITY

MMA is an excellent way to improve health and lose weight, and many people become involved in the sport for this reason. Research shows that individuals who are overweight and physically active are significantly less likely to develop cardiovascular disease than thin, inactive people. You do not have to look like one of the people on the front of an MMA magazine to be healthy. There are certain key points you should consider when training MMA while overweight or obese.

If you are overweight you are much more susceptible to the development of heat-related injuries, as fat storage acts as insulation, reducing the body's ability to effectively dissipate heat. While this can be beneficial on cold days, it is counterproductive on hot, humid days. Many gyms can get really hot in the summer, and you should be cognizant of signs and symptoms of heat-related illness when training.

Running is a training tool commonly used to increase the aerobic capacity of fighters. Keep in mind that running is a weight-bearing activity, and the impact (ground reaction forces) is two to three times your body weight. Due to impact and body weight, it is important to begin the running session of your program slowly, listen to your body, and make adjustments accordingly. Beginning at too high a volume or intensity may result in the development of overuse injuries, for example, stress fractures or joint injuries. It is normal to feel slight discomfort, but you should not feel pain during a run. The development of sharp pains is a sign of possible damage and should be evaluated by a physician. You may even want to begin your aerobic program with activities that are non-weight-bearing, for instance, cycling. This will give you the aerobic improvements without undue stress on the joints. You can add in running later as you progress.

DIABETES

Diagnosed diabetics are typically well versed on their disease, treatment, and symptoms. While you may be confident that you can manage your diabetes, you should still consult with your doctor when beginning a training program for MMA. This section is not intended to provide medical advice, but instead discuss a few key considerations that you may wish to discuss with your doctor. When developing a plan with your doctor, talk about how to alter diet and insulin injections, if needed, to accommodate your current level of training.

Another reason for obtaining a physician's clearance prior to starting a training program is that diabetes can result in the development of other health complications. Some of the common comorbidities are high blood pressure, cardiovascular disease, compromised peripheral vascularization, and peripheral neuropathy. While exercise is recommended for individuals with diabetes, it is important that diabetes is under control prior to starting a program and that control is maintained throughout training. Once cleared to participate in physical activity, you must monitor blood glucose levels before, during, and after training and adjust accordingly.

Diabetics are well versed in the pathophysiology of diabetes and related factors. The following information is more for the coaches and trainers who may be working with diabetics. While there are other pathologies, I will discuss the two basic pathologies for the occurrence of diabetes. The first pathology occurs when the insulin-producing cells located on the pancreas are damaged, which ultimately limits insulin production. This usually occurs due to an autoimmune dysfunction where the body's immune system attacks the cells. Because the pancreas cannot produce adequate amounts of insulin, many diabetics will need to inject insulin into their system. This type of diabetes is typically referred to as type I, or early onset, diabetes.

Whereas type I diabetes is a result of a decrease in insulin production, type II diabetes is a result of a decrease in insulin sensitivity at the insulin receptor cites. Insulin receptor sites are downregulated (a reduction in hormone receptor sites) in response to chronic high levels of insulin being released into the system. This commonly occurs due to an overabundance of foods that are high on the glycemic index, resulting in regular insulin spikes to offset spikes in blood glucose. The two primary risk factors for the development of type II diabetes are being sedentary and being overweight.

Both exercise and proper diet have a strong effect on both type I and type II diabetes. Because of permanent damage to the islet beta cells of the pancreas, exercise and proper diet do not provide a cure for type I diabetes; however, a combination of exercise and diet can positively impact type I diabetes, helping keep the disease more controlled. Diet and exercise have a much stronger impact on type II diabetes, as they increase insulin sensitivity.

If you have diabetes, work with a registered dietitian who is familiar with sport performance. It is unlikely that the average coach will have sufficient knowledge to adequately assess and prescribe proper nutrition to a diabetic, and some state regulations even prohibit giving nutritional advice to those with diabetes.

Low blood sugar (hypoglycemia) is of great concern for diabetic athletes, which is why it is important to monitor blood glucose levels before, during, and after exercise. Glycogen (the storage form of blood sugar) and glucose are the only sources of energy the brain can use; therefore, when blood glucose levels are low, the brain and central nervous systems are negatively impacted. The initial response to low blood sugar is the release of epinephrine (commonly referred to as adrenaline) in an attempt to increase blood sugar. The release of epinephrine results in a significant increase in heart rate, the development of muscle tremors, anxiety, and an increased appetite. These are the most common early warning symptoms of hypoglycemia. As hypoglycemia begins to affect the brain, symptoms of hypoglycemia worsen, resulting in headache, dizziness, fatigue, irritability, slurred speech, blurred vision, confusion, lack of coordination, and unconsciousness. In severe cases, hypoglycemia can even result in coma or death.

Hypoglycemia can progress quickly, and training should cease instantly upon the presentation of symptoms. The fighter should immediately measure blood glucose and respond accordingly. Diabetic athletes will typically keep foods high on the glycemic index available to help counteract a hypoglycemic episode. The athlete should eat, recheck blood sugar levels, and make an educated decision about whether to continue training. If blood sugar levels are not within the normal limits or the athlete does not feel well, the training session should be canceled.

Training for MMA places a heavy strain on glycogen stores and blood glucose levels; therefore, adjustments to both diet and insulin may need to be considered. It is important to remember that blood glucose is released from the liver and into the blood at a much higher rate during anaerobic bouts. Insulin-dependent fighters may need to adjust insulin timing and dosage. Diabetic fighters who use an insulin pump need to take this into consideration when training and competing, as there is risk of the insertion site becoming loose. There are two common options used in combat sports. The most common option is to switch to injections during competition. The next option is to switch the insertion site to the leg and underneath compression shorts, and disconnect the pump during the match. You will need to check with the commissioning body to see if this option is allowed during competition. This is not medical advice;

I am simply stating that these are two commonly used methods. It is important that you do not make any alterations to your diet or timing, delivery system, or dosage of insulin before thoroughly discussing it with your physician prior to implementation.

Cutting to make weight can be difficult and could lead to negative health consequences for diabetics. It is recommended that you compete as close to your walk-around weight as possible. Alterations to diet to drop weight can result in unhealthy alterations to blood glucose levels. Always consult with your doctor prior to making drastic changes to your diet.

ASTHMA

Asthma is characterized by difficulty breathing, and it is one of the most common chronic diseases that affects athletes. During an asthma attack the air passage constricts and mucus builds up, interfering with normal breathing. The severity of asthma attacks varies and ranges from slight discomfort while breathing to a life-threatening blockage. For some athletes, asthma only occurs in relation to physical exertion, where an episode will occur only during or shortly after exercise and is known as exercise-induced asthma. It is important to note that asthmatic symptoms can present 5 to 10 minutes after the cessation of exercise. Any asthma trigger (pollen, carbon monoxide, etc.) can increase the risk of exercise-induced asthma. Environmental factors also play a role. Cold, dry environments greatly increase the risk of an incident, whereas warm, humid environments reduce the risk.

A slow, gradual, and longer warm-up is recommended for those diagnosed with asthma. If you have frequent or severe asthma, pay close attention to your warm-up protocol. If prescribed by a physician, an inhaler can be used prior to competition to help prevent an occurrence. Never train without your inhaler physically present. As a coach, it is always a good idea to have the athlete show their inhaler prior to the start of any session. Inhalers contain banned substances (primarily albuterol); therefore, use of an inhaler requires a medical waiver.

DISABLED ATHLETES

Learning MMA is an excellent idea for everyone, and disabilities should not discourage or eliminate anyone from pursuing the sport. For the context of this discussion, disabilities will be all-encompassing, covering everything from physical and intellectual diseases to neuromuscular diseases. Both fighting and strength and conditioning techniques can be adapted to accommodate an athlete's individual disability. You can find numerous examples of disabled athletes who have been successful in combat sports. It is beyond the scope of this book to give detailed advice for specific disabilities, so instead I will focus on general advice for those with disabilities.

The first important step is to know and understand your specific disability as it relates to physical activity. Adjustments in technique will need to be made to accommodate for your specific disability. Do not get stuck in the trap of trying to precisely follow the taught techniques when your disability prevents you from doing so. It will be frustrating and nonproductive. Instead, focus on the idea of the technique and what that technique is supposed to accomplish. Once you understand the desired outcome, the next step is to develop a technique to accommodate for your disability that produces the same desired outcome. This is true for any physical activity whether it be MMA, lifting, or running.

MMA is not a sport without a related risk of injury. Some sports do possess greater risk than others, and MMA is high on that list. Depending on your disability you may or may not be at greater risk than the average athlete; therefore, it is important to understand your specific disability-related risks when it comes to participating in MMA. Speak with your doctor about your desire to become involved in MMA and discuss any specific concerns for participation, increased risks of participation, and adaptations that need to be made for you to safely and effectively participate. After speaking with your doctor make a list of concerns, risks, and necessary adaptations, and discuss this list with your coach so you can develop a strong plan.

Educate your coach about your disability. He may have never coached an athlete with your specific disability, and the more knowledge they have the better they can assist you in reaching your goals. It is important to not only educate them about your specific disability, but also let them know you are not made of glass. You are there to participate to the fullest of your ability and want to be challenged and learn and grow just like anyone else they coach.

Lastly, there are many organizations that work with disabled athletes. The International Paralympic Committee is a great resource for disabled athletes (https://www.paralympic.org/). While they do not currently have MMA as a sport, they do have judo and taekwondo. There are many other organizations that offer training and information for disabled athletes. These organizations provide not only information, but also an opportunity for you to connect with other athletes who have similar disabilities and are willing to share their experiences. Reach out and find an organization that best fits your personal situation.

8

INJURY AND INJURY PREVENTION IN MIXED MARTIAL ARTS

This chapter is designed to provide basic information on injury and injury prevention in mixed martial arts (MMA). MMA is a high-risk sport where injuries are very common in both training and competition. Many of the injuries that occur during participation in MMA will require medical attention and follow-up medical advice, and therefore are not covered in detail in this chapter. Some of those common injuries are dental, lacerations, fractures, dislocations, concussions, and muscular tears. This chapter focuses on injuries for which there are preventable measures that can be taken. I will discuss both the mechanism of the injury and any possible injury prevention strategies. The following is not meant to be medical advice, and you should always be evaluated by a doctor when an injury occurs.

PHYSICAL EXAM

When starting an MMA program, it is important that you obtain a physical exam to ensure that you are healthy enough to participate. If you have been inactive up to this point, it is even more important to have a physical exam prior to starting MMA, as being sedentary is a major risk factor for the development of cardiovascular disease, type II diabetes, high cholesterol, high blood pressure, and other medical problems. A physical exam will catch medical conditions that you may not be aware you have.

If you have a diagnosed disease state, doctors will often recommend physical activity as a method for improvement of overall health and daily activities. If you are currently under the care of a doctor for a specific disease state, it is important that you consult with your doctor prior to participating in MMA. They will be in the best position to advise you on your involvement in the sport.

It is recommended that older individuals (males older than 45 and females older than 55) should seek medical clearance prior to beginning any exercise program. As we age, we become more susceptible to the development of specific disease states, for example, cardiovascular disease. As MMA is a high-intensity contact sport, it is vital that older individuals seek medical clearance prior to beginning a program.

If you have any signs or symptoms of cardiovascular disease you should seek medical clearance prior to participating in an MMA program. The following is a list of the common signs/symptoms associated with cardiovascular disease. This is not an all-inclusive list, and the signs/symptoms only indicate the possibility of cardiovascular disease. Only your physician can diagnose it or rule it out. Also, keep in mind that cardiovascular disease can be asymptomatic. Some of the signs and symptoms are as follows:

- Chest pain at rest or during exercise
- Pain in the arms, shoulder, neck, or jaw regions
- Abnormal shortness of breath
- Irregular heartbeat (speed or rhythm)
- Edema in the ankles
- Cramping in the calf muscles
- Unusual fatigue
- Dizziness
- Fainting
- Difficulty breathing when lying down

When looking for a primary physician, I always recommend finding a sport-specific doctor or at least a physician who understands athletes. They will have a better understanding of the stress you will be putting your body through and the mind-set that goes along with being a fighter. I have found better results when working with a physician who understands how the body responds to training and has a strong understanding of the athlete mind-set.

When suffering from muscular injuries, connective tissue damage, or bone damage, I recommend seeking medical advice from an orthopedic sports medicine specialist. These practitioners have a strong background in sports medicine, giving them insight into the mechanisms behind the injury and what it will take to optimally get you back to training and competing. They can make better decisions about your training load and what you can and cannot handle given your specific situation.

ILLNESS

Overall, exercise is good for the body and results in improved immune function in healthy individuals; however, a hard training session actually challenges the immune system, making you more susceptible to developing an illness just after the completion of training. Athletes who train correctly will have improved immune function compared to sedentary individuals; however, athletes who are frequently overtrained have compromised immune function. Frequent or persistent illness is a common sign of overtraining.

There are a few general guidelines to follow for training when ill. In most cases, training should be avoided when you do not feel well, as your illness may become worse or last longer than it otherwise would have. Training should be avoided if you feel nauseous; have a fever, headache, and/or body aches; or experience severe fatigue. In most cases you are okay to train with a cold as long as you do not have a fever, body aches, or chest congestion.

When your immune system is already fighting an illness, you do not want to lower its ability to perform by exercising. Missing a few days of training to recover from an illness will not completely derail your training program, whereas attempting to push through an illness could make it worse and result in increased time off from training.

When taking over-the-counter or prescribed medicine it is important to know how the medication can interact with exercise. For example, decongestants can act as a stimulant, resulting in a significant increase in resting and submaximal heart rate. While this may not be harmful, it can result in alteration to training zones while on decongestants. Decongestants can also result in dehydration and drowsiness. Always ask your doctor how your medication can affect exercise.

CONCUSSIONS

Concussions are not uncommon in MMA and typically occur due to a strike landing to the head or contact with the mat during a takedown. Concussions can cause permanent noticeable damage either acutely (one event) or chronically (a massed effect of multiple concussions) and should be taken seriously. Throughout time repeated damage to the brain from fighting can result in dementia pugilistica (boxer's dementia), where there is a significant loss in cognitive function. The prevalence of concussions in combat sports has understandably resulted in increased research on concussion treatment and prevention. While I am discussing concussions, keep in mind that you do not have to have a "notice-able" concussion to experience brain damage.

Concussions occur when the brain accelerates and makes contact with the side of the skull, causing damage. The whip-like motion also results in damage to the brain, nerve axons, and blood vessels. When blood vessels are ruptured, bleeding and edema occurs in the brain. Subdural hematomas (bleeding of the brain), which occur when blood vessels are damaged due to an impact, are the most common cause of death in combat sports (MMA, boxing, Muay Thai, etc.). Strikes that cause the head to accelerate in a rotational fashion will cause the most damage and have a higher likelihood of resulting in a knockout. Straight-line blows will cause damage but are less likely to cause a knockout compared to blows that cause rotation.

It is important to recognize the symptoms of concussion, as your brain is more susceptible to greater damage while concussed. The most common symptoms of concussion are the following:

- Headache
- Dizziness
- Trouble focusing/confusion
- Blurred vision
- Nausea
- Ringing in the ears
- Slurred speech
- Memory loss
- Unconsciousness (you do not have to experience unconsciousness to have a concussion)
- Uncoordinated movements

If you are diagnosed with a concussion, it is important that you are cleared by a doctor prior to returning to MMA. You are more susceptible to further brain injury when recovering from a concussion. A concussion can also interfere with your balance, cognitive abilities, and motor control, resulting in poor physical performance, which has the consequence of you getting hit more often.

There are a few methods you can use to decrease the risk of concussion and head trauma. One of the most important methods is to reduce the number of times you spar hard. You can gain a lot of skill and experience when sparring lighter, and there is no need to spar hard every time you spar. Keep in mind that brain damage can occur chronically throughout time due to numerous small injuries, as well as from one large impact. I will not spar with individuals who do not understand or refuse to use control when sparring. You will quickly learn who to spar with at your gym and who you should steer clear from. It is also important that you set the tone of the sparring match prior to starting and stick with it throughout. If you want an easy sparring session, you need to state that fact prior to the session, and do not allow it to escalate. Call someone out if they say they are going to go easy and then come out swinging. Do not let them dictate the level, and walk away when needed. There will be times when you accidentally strike someone too hard due to bad timing or your opponent coming forward as you throw the strike. When this occurs, apologize, make sure they are good, and deescalate the situation.

Another method is to make sure that you are using well-padded and soft gloves during sparring. Do not be afraid to tell someone when they need new gloves, and check yours regularly, as gloves wear out. I have a good heavy pair of gel gloves that I use for heavy bag and pad work, and I have a second set of 16-ounce soft leather gloves that I use for sparring.

Use of headgear to prevent brain injury is somewhat controversial at this point, as mentioned earlier in this book. Headgear can be useful in preventing brain injuries if used in the correct manner. Keep in mind that headgear is not an invitation to hit harder, as it does not provide the protection you believe it does. Even with headgear, you should go light, and remember, the headgear is only there for when a strike is accidentally miscalculated or your opponent moves into your strike. Headgear can also decrease peripheral vision, resulting in taking more hits. Choose headgear with good padding and peripheral vision to reduce the number of blows.

ANTERIOR CRUCIATE LIGAMENT

The anterior cruciate ligament (ACL) is attached to the femur and tibia, and used to provide anterior stability to the knee. The ACL is commonly injured during contact sports and sports that have strong cutting motions. During MMA, there are two primary mechanisms that commonly result in ACL tears. The first mechanism involves the foot being planted and the knee twisting. This situation can occur when you are moving around the ring and changing directions, twisting of the knee during groundwork, or rotating on your planted foot as you throw a kick. The second mechanism for ACL injuries involves direct force applied to the knee through such common tactics as knee kicks or movements, for example, a knee lock. ACL tears can put a fighter out of commission for an extended period of time for surgery and recovery. Gender also plays a factor, as females are six to eight times more likely to develop an ACL injury compared to their male counterparts due to biomechanical gender differences.

There are a few methods you can use to reduce the risk of ACL injury. The first is to work on strengthening muscles of the lower extremities. The stronger the joint, the less likely it will subluxate or dislocate. The second is to offset any strength discrepancies between the quadriceps and hamstrings. It is common that the quadricep muscles will be significantly stronger than the hamstring muscles. This causes a greater anterior pull on the knee and greater stress on the ACL. Increasing the strength of the hamstring muscles offsets this discrepancy and increases the stability of the knee. Improving agility and balance will also assist in dynamic knee stability. While none of these factors will eliminate the risk of an ACL injury, they will significantly reduce the risk.

MAT BURN AND GI BURN

Mat burns and gi burns are common when training MMA. Mat burns occur due to friction created between your skin and the mat. The wound left by mat burn is partially an abrasion and partially a burn due to heat from the friction. Mat burns are less common when flow rolling and increase in occurrence as intensity increases. One of the best ways to avoid mat burn is to make sure your skin is covered. When wearing a jiujitsu gi, the majority of your skin is covered; however, in no-gi rolling you have more skin exposed. This is why wearing a rash guard during no-gi rolling is extremely important. The feet and toes are a common area of concern, as they are not covered when rolling and subject to frequent mat burns. Throughout time the skin of your feet and toes will toughen up, and mat burn will become less of an issue. When you have mat burn on your toes or feet you can use bandages and athletic tape until the wound heals to prevent infection or further mat burn to that area while it is already damaged.

Gi burns can occur anywhere the gi touches your skin but typically occur around the neck and face area from gi chokes. Gi burns typically only occur during heavy rolls. To prevent gi burns, it is recommended to wear a rash guard under your gi. One of the best ways to prevent gi burns around the face and neck is to learn proper gi choke defense and tap during training when you feel the gi burning across your neck or face. Always remember that it is just training, and nothing is on the line at that point. Save it for competition.

Mat burns are open wounds and, as such, very susceptible to infection. Even the best-cleaned mats hold the potential for infection. Clean the wound to remove any debris, apply an antibacterial ointment, and keep it covered as it is healing. Before your next training session make sure that you put antibacterial ointment on the wound, bandage it, and use enough athletic tape so that the bandage does not come off while rolling. Keep an eye on the wound. and look for any signs of infection. Some common signs of infection are the following:

- Swelling
- Increased pain
- Wound enlargement
- Spreading redness around the wound
- Fever
- Puss and drainage

If infection is suspected, seek medical aid immediately.

COMMON SKIN INFECTIONS

Unfortunately, skin infections are not uncommon in MMA. I will discuss a few of the more common skin infections you may be exposed to during your MMA training. If you have a suspected skin infection, the best thing you can do is go to the doctor immediately. The earlier you treat skin infections the faster they will heal and the less damage they can do.

The first skin infection I will discuss is a fungal infection called tinea. Tinea can grow anywhere on the body and is identified by different nomenclature depending on the area of the body where the fungus presents. When the fungus presents on the feet it is known as athlete's foot, in the groin area it is known as jock itch, and anywhere else on the body it is known as ringworm.

Athlete's foot appears on the foot and toes, and is extremely itchy. The skin will be red and flaky, and may peel and blister. Jock itch presents the same as athlete's foot but in the groin area. Ringworm presents as an itchy patch on the skin with a red circle and lighter middle, which is how the fungal infection received the name. Ringworm presents on the scalp in a similar fashion but can look like an irritated pimple.

If tinea is expected, visit the doctor and take care of the fungus early before it spreads. If caught early, most cases can be treated with a topical antifungal, but if it spreads the fungus will need to be treated with internal medicine. Make sure to keep the area clean and dry, as fungal infections thrive in wet areas.

Staphylococcus aureus (commonly referred to as staph) is a bacterial infection that is transferred through open or damaged skin. Staph infections typically are not serious as long as they are caught and treated early before the infection enters deeper into the body. If the infection enters the bloodstream it can become serious. Methicillin-resistant staphylococcus aureus (MRSA) is a strain of staph infection that is resistant to antibiotics and can be hard to fight. If a staph infection is suspected seek medical attention immediately. Staph infections can present as follows:

- Boils
- Blisters
- Skin abscesses
- Cellulitis
- Red irritated skin
- Puss and drainage
- Tenderness
- Fever and illness with serious infections

Treatment for staph infections varies with the type and seriousness of the infection, and medical treatment is strongly recommended. As untreated staph infections can become deadly, the earlier you catch the infection and begin treatment the better off you will be.

Herpes gladiatorum is a term used to define the viral infection herpes simplex type I for combative athletes. It is commonly referred to as mat herpes. The virus is easily transferred when the carrier has open lesions, and once an individual contracts herpes, they will carry the virus for life. Skin-to-skin contact is the most common form of transfer in combat sports. Symptoms of mat herpes are the following:

- Sores on the skin
- Blisters on the skin
- Fever
- Sore throat
- Headache
- Swollen glands

Prevention of Common Skin Infections

While skin infections are not 100 percent preventable there are steps you can take to reduce the risk of developing one. Here are a few steps you can take:

- Never step onto the mat with an open wound that is not covered.
- Never train with someone who has an uncovered open wound. Ask your partner to cover their wounds or simply do not train with them.
- Wash your training clothes regularly and thoroughly, as bacteria thrive in damp, dirty areas. Training in dirty, unwashed clothing puts you and your training partners at risk.
- Remove your training clothes and shower as soon as possible upon completion of training. Sitting around in damp, dirty gear provides an ideal breeding ground for bacteria.
- Clean your training gear on a regular basis. Boxing gloves, shin guards, and so on are excellent environments for the growth of bacteria.
- Ensure that where you train maintains a well-sanitized training area. Mats and equipment (heavy bags, Thai pads, etc.) should be cleaned between each class block and at the end of the night.
- Every gym has a standing rule that you should not train if you are contagious. Make sure you and your training partners always follow this rule. Do not hide any skin rashes.
- Clip and file smooth both fingernails and toenails. This prevents the transfer of bacteria and the loss of willing training partners.
- Do not store clothing or equipment in your gym bag. It is okay to transfer equipment to and from training in a gym bag; however, once you are home immediately remove all gear for cleaning.

OVERUSE INJURIES

Unfortunately, overuse injuries are quite common in MMA. The sport requires repetitive motions that place stress on the muscles, connective tissue, bones, and joint structure. An overuse injury presents as chronic pain in a specific area that is directly related to training. An overuse injury can hurt before, during, and after training. Some overuse injuries may feel fine during training but then hurt after training or the next day when you get out of bed (plantar fasciitis is an example). The pain can range from mild and annoying to excruciating. If not addressed appropriately the damage and pain can increase with continued training. Persistent pain should be evaluated by a doctor.

There are many factors that can attribute to overuse injuries. Many of these factors relate to improper training. One of the common mistakes made by beginning mixed martial artists is that they increase volume or intensity too quickly. Remember to progress your training in a controlled and correctly paced manner. Always increase your volume first and then your intensity once you establish a solid base.

Another common cause of overuse injury is overtraining. It is important that you allow adequate recovery time between training bouts. When you ignore recovery and do not allow adequate recovery between bouts it leaves the body in a weakened state and susceptible to the development of an overuse injury. This is especially true when your program contains two-a-day training sessions. Be as diligent about your recovery as you are about your training.

Lack of flexibility is another leading cause of overuse injury in MMA. I cannot count the number of athletes I have worked with whose overuse injuries were the result of lack of flexibility. Once the flexibility issues were addressed, the overuse injury subsided. When joints are not able to easily go through their full range of motion during exercise, it can result in strain in that area and the development of an overuse injury. MMA requires good flexibility to correctly move through the required range of motion for fighting techniques. Throwing high kicks at the limit of your flexibility will lead to incorrect form and can result in overuse injuries.

Muscular strength around a joint can also play a factor in the development of overuse injuries. The weaker the muscles around a joint, the less stable that joint is and the more susceptible to the development of an overuse injury. Muscular imbalances can also lead to the development of an overuse injury. For example, if the quadriceps muscles are significantly stronger than the hamstring muscles, it will result in an anterior pull at the knee, resulting in static and dynamic instability. The closer the match in strength between the hamstring and the quadriceps muscles, the more stable the joint will be. You should work on not only increasing strength, but also ensuring muscular balance.

Repetitive mechanical loads can result in overuse injuries. This scenario most often occurs in MMA from heavy bag workouts and presents as sore shoulders, wrists, thumbs, or knuckles. The common mechanisms are hitting too hard, too often; improper form; and improper protection. To limit overuse injuries from heavy bag workouts it is important that you protect your hands. Make sure you are using quality gloves with good padding and that your hands are wrapped appropriately. Ensure that you are working out on a quality bag. A bag that is low quality or worn out can be hard on your body. Replace both your gloves and the heavy bag as they wear out. Make sure you are performing your strikes properly so that they land correctly on the bag. Lastly, do not strike the heavy bag all out every time you train. Instead make sure that you slow down and focus on technique only on occasion.

The last primary cause of overuse injuries is improper biomechanics or technique. For each punch or kick there is a correct movement pattern that must be performed to ensure that the strike is both effective and safe. Improper striking techniques can result in undue stress placed on the joints of the arms and legs. The shoulder, elbow, and wrist are often injured due to improperly thrown punches. Improperly thrown kicks can result in knee damage as well. Spend time with your coach to ensure you have the proper biomechanics down.

As you will be implementing resistance training in your MMA program it is important that you learn the correct techniques for each lift and movement you will be using. Improper resistance techniques is one of the primary reasons for overuse injuries when lifting.

Shoulder Pain

Shoulder pain is not uncommon in MMA, as the shoulders are often used when punching and during groundwork. The muscles of the rotator cuff are designed to maintain static and dynamic stability of the humeral head within the glenoid fossa. Keep in mind that the muscles of the rotator cuff are small and easily fatigued. As the muscles and ligaments of the shoulder become loose, the shoulder can subluxate, leading to tendinitis and muscular damage. To help prevent overuse injuries of the shoulder it is important to work on muscular strength and endurance to strengthen the muscles around the shoulder joint. Muscular imbalances also need to be addressed. Make sure you develop a well-balanced program. Also, keep in mind that there are a lot of different mechanisms for shoulder pain, and it could be anything from impingement, to tendinitis, to a torn labrum, to a torn rotator cuff muscle. Persistent pain should be evaluated by a doctor. This is especially true if you have pronounced weakness in the joint, as well as pain.

Knee Pain

Knee pain can occur in MMA due to footwork drills, running, and jumping. Knee pain is often referred to as "runner's knee," even though you are not a "runner." This term is frequently used as a catchall for any pain that occurs in the area of the knee while running. By this definition, there are any number of issues that could be occurring. When medical professionals discuss runner's knee it is specific to the anterior portion of the knee centered around the patella. There are two common pathologies that result in anterior knee pain centered around the patella. The first involves pain centered directly behind the patella. This pain is most often the result of improper tracking of the patella and undue pressure on the patella as it passes across the femur. This scenario can result in the development of chondromalacia (deterioration of cartilage on the posterior patella). The second common pathology is pain along the patellar tendon (patella tendonitis). Common causes of runner's knee are muscular weaknesses, muscular imbalances, patella tracking issues, and repetitive strain placed on the knee while running.

Constant knee pain should be evaluated by a doctor to ensure that you are not causing greater damage by continuing to train. There are a few steps you can take to help alleviate the problem. The first is to ensure that you are running in good running shoes that fit you correctly. Another is to strengthen the muscles around the joint to increase stability of the joint area and possibly help with any patella tracking issues. Increase your flexibility so you can comfortably go through the full range of motion at each joint. Pay close attention to the hamstrings and glutes, as this is where most runners are tight and do not realize that they are.

Plantar Fasciitis

Plantar fasciitis presents as pain along the bottom of the foot located at the heel. Plantar fasciitis can be very painful. The plantar fascia is the connective tissue that runs along the bottom of the foot from the calcaneus of the heel to the toes and is responsible for maintaining the longitudinal arch of the foot. Plantar fasciitis occurs when the plantar fascia becomes damaged and inflamed. While damage can occur acutely, it often takes place due to repeated stress. Pain occurs when training but can worsen after a training session. Plantar fasciitis can be very painful when you get out of bed in the morning or if you have been in a stationary period for a prolonged period of time, for instance, sitting at a desk. This soreness occurs due to the plantar fascia shortening and tightening. It is not uncommon for the pain to decrease throughout the day as the fascia loosens up as you move around. It is often recommended to sleep in a night splint, keeping the foot in a neutral position and the fascia from shortening and tightening too much during the night. When running, the large ground reaction forces place a heavy strain on the plantar fascia. Plantar fasciitis is common in individuals with abnormal arches (too high or too low). Plantar fasciitis is typically caused by long runs, excessive downhill running, and lack of flexibility.

Achilles Tendinitis

Achilles tendinitis presents as a pain located in the Achilles tendon. When running and jumping, the triceps surae (gastrocnemius and soleus) is used heavily during plantar flexion of the toe off phase. The triceps surae attaches to the posterior surface of the calcaneus via the Achilles tendon. Plantar flexion during running and jumping places a lot of strain on the Achilles tendon and can lead to Achilles tendinopathy. This condition is most commonly caused by too high an intensity or volume, lack of general flexibility, poor biomechanics, heavy uphill running, or jumping rope.

Iliotibial Band Syndrome

The tensor fascia latae originates on the iliac crest, runs downward on the lateral side of the leg, and ties into the iliotibial band (IT band), which inserts on the Gerdy's tubercle of the tibia. The IT band is a thick fascia of connective tissue that makes up most of the length from the iliac crest to the tibia. It is important that you can visualize the muscle to better understand IT band syndrome. The tensor fascia latae is used heavily in running, as it is responsible for ensuring that the leg swings forward in a straight manner. The gluteus maximus places a large amount of strain on the IT band when running, since it is used heavily during hip extension. To help avoid or eliminate IT band syndrome, work on hip and IT band flexibility.

It is important to address overuse injuries early on to prevent greater damage. Too often athletes will ignore overuse injuries until they develop into an injury that requires a large amount of downtime or surgery. If you develop an overuse injury it is important that you address it seriously. If the pain is sharp or persistent, have it evaluated by a doctor. A common practice with most overuse injuries is to use rest, ice, and elevation. When approved by your doctor, over-the-counter antiinflammatory medications can help decrease swelling and alleviate pain.

EXERCISING IN THE HEAT

Training in the heat places a great amount of strain on the human body. Heat is generated as a byproduct of metabolism. As intensity increases, so too does metabolism, resulting in an increase in internal temperature. This internal heat generation during exercise, coupled with environmental heat, creates a very precarious situation.

The two methods of heat entering the body from the environment during training are radiation and conduction. Radiation is the primary method and is the transfer of heat through electromagnetic waves. The sun provides radiant heat and is the most common form. Radiation from the sun can be either direct or reflected off objects, for example, asphalt. During the summer, thermal ground heat will radiate upward and can be transferred to the body during training. Conduction is not experienced to a large degree during training, as it requires direct molecular contact for heat to transfer. The most common form of conduction during training is when the foot makes contact with the hot ground.

To prevent a heat-related illness, it is important to dissipate heat effectively from the body. For the body to dissipate heat through radiation, the body temperature must be higher than the environmental temperature. Conduction is not an effective method for heat dissipation during exercise either; therefore, the two main sources for heat dissipation during exercise are convection and evaporation. Convection is the transfer of heat through a fluid medium. As the air travels across the body, the boundary layer of air next to the skin is continuously replaced with cooler air. The faster the boundary layer is replaced, the faster the body can dissipate heat. This is how fans work to help keep the body cool during exercise.

Evaporation of sweat on the skin transfers heat to the environment and is the primary method of heat dissipation during exercise. For the cooling process to occur, the sweat must evaporate on the skin. Relative humidity (the ratio of water contained in the air compared to the amount the air could contain) affects the ability of the human body to cool through the use of evaporation. If the relative humidity is 60 percent, then 40 percent of the air can accept the water. If the relative humidity is 90 percent, then only 10 percent of the air can absorb water, leaving little room for evaporation to occur and negatively impacting evaporative cooling during exercise. Windy days are beneficial, as air moving across the skin will continually replace the boundary layer with less saturated air to aid in cooling.

During exercise, heat is generated by the working muscles, increasing both muscle and core temperature. For cooling to occur, the heat must be transferred from the muscles and core to the skin so that it can be dissipated into the surrounding environment. Blood makes an excellent transporter of heat, as roughly 50 to 55 percent of the blood consists of water. Autoregulation of blood flow allows for the redirection of blood flow to the skin to dissipate heat through evaporation, convection, and radiation. The cooled blood will then recirculate back through the body to pick up more heat, and the process repeats. Keep in mind that as heat increases, a greater amount of blood flow will be redirected to the skin. This lowers the volume of blood flow to the working muscles and reduces performance.

As you can see, blood is vital in the process of heat dissipation. As blood is made up of predominantly water, hydration status strongly impacts the body's ability to cool. When you become dehydrated, your ability to cool the body is strongly impacted. To make a long story short, sweat is filtered plasma, and as you sweat plasma volume decreases. The decrease in plasma volume results in dehydration and impaired cooling. As your ability to dissipate heat becomes compromised, the core temperature begins to steadily rise, resulting in the development of a heat-related illness. Water loss equivalent to 2 to 3 percent of body mass will negatively impact performance, whereas a loss equivalent to 5 percent or greater will negatively impact health. These numbers assume that you began the session fully hydrated.

Heat-Related Illness

Heat-related illness occurs when the body's ability to dissipate heat has been compromised due to high internal and external temperatures, as well as dehydration. Heat-related illness is of serious concern and can result in death if untreated. As a fighter there are many discomforts or pains you can push through (I do not advise this course of action); however, a heat related illness is not one of them. The primary heat-related illnesses are heat cramps, heat exhaustion, and heat stroke.

Heat Cramps

Heat cramps present as strong and painful muscle contractions that occur due to dehydration and sodium loss. The best way to counter heat cramps is to stop exercising, get to a cool environment, rehydrate, and ingest electrolytes.

Heat Exhaustion

As your ability to dissipate heat continues to diminish, the thermoregulatory system is unable to effectively dissipate heat. The primary symptoms of heat exhaustion are as follows:

- Headache
- Dizziness

- Nausea
- Weakness
- Tingling sensation in the skin
- Chills
- Pale, moist skin
- Rapid, weak pulse

Heat Stroke

As you progress beyond heat exhaustion, your ability to further dissipate heat could result in heat stroke. Of the three heat-related illnesses, heat stroke is the worst, as it can cause serious health issues, including death. Some of the heat stroke symptoms are the same as those found in heat exhaustion. There are a few key symptoms that differ, the most important of which is the development of a core temperature of 104° F or higher. The other differing symptoms are cessation of sweating and hot, red, dry skin, as signs that you have moved from heat exhaustion to heat stroke. The following is a full list of the symptoms of heat stroke:

- Core temperature greater than or equal to 104° F
- Hot, red, dry skin
- Cessation of sweating
- Rapid, strong pulse
- Headache
- Dizziness
- Nausea
- Weakness
- Tingling sensation in the skin
- Confusion
- Chills

At the first sign of a heat-related illness, you should stop exercising immediately, cool the body down as quickly as possible, and drink plenty of fluids. As heat-related injuries can escalate in severity in a very quick progression, it is important to cease activity immediately at the first sign. Once core temperature starts to increase beyond the body's ability to control it, it will continue to rise as long as you exercise and generate metabolic heat in a hot environment.

Once you have ceased activity and moved into a cooler environment, continue working to bring the core temperature down. There are methods you can use to lower core temperature to normal levels, for instance, taking a cool shower or bath, applying cold towels, or using ice packs. As dehydration is a key component of heat-related illness, it is also important to ingest fluids. Rehydration can become problematic when you are nauseous and cannot keep fluids down. If this is the case, a trip to the doctor and an IV will most likely be required. If you suspect that you have heat stroke, seek medical attention immediately.

Prevention

The best way to deal with heat-related illness is to not have an event in the first place. What follows are a few basic prevention strategies that will help you avoid heat-related illness. When training outside avoid the hottest part of the day and instead train early, before the temperatures get too high. If training indoors, try to keep the temperature as cool as possible, and use fans.

Choose appropriate clothing when training in the heat. Clothing should be breathable so sweat is able to evaporate on the skin to cool the body. When training outside, do not wear dark colors, as they will absorb radiation from the sun to a much greater extent than lighter colors.

As stated earlier, proper hydration is important for dissipating heat and maintaining a functioning core temperature. Unfortunately, most athletes are chronically dehydrated during the summertime due to long hours training and inadequate hydration strategies. Keep track of water loss and ingestion to help maintain proper hydration levels. Weigh yourself before and after training to determine water loss, and replace each pound lost with approximately 24 ounces of fluid.

Acclimatization is the strongest step you can take to help prevent heat-related illness. It will take approximately two weeks of training in the heat for significant physiological changes to occur during the acclimatization process. As the body adapts to the heat, more blood will be directed to the skin for cooling, and there will be a more efficient distribution of blood throughout the body. There will be significant alterations to sweating; you will begin to sweat more, sweat will start at a lower core temperature, and sweat will be better distributed on the body to optimize cooling. Sodium concentrations in sweat will decrease to help offset electrolyte imbalances that occur during heavy sodium loss. Glycogen use significantly increases when exercising in the heat. After acclimation, glycogen use will not be as high as prior to acclimation. This will spare glycogen stores, which are limited and can negatively impact performance when diminished.

To appropriately acclimate to training in the heat you will want to start slowly and during cooler parts of the day. Do not attempt to acclimate by training during the hottest parts of the day or conducting high-volume or high-intensity workouts in the heat. Instead, start increasing volume and intensity after a minimum two-week acclimation period.

INDEX

ABOUT THE AUTHOR

Will Peveler is a noted physiologist with a teaching and research focus on physiological and biomechanical factors that influence sport performance. He works as professor of exercise science at Liberty University. Peveler has a strong background in martial arts and continues to train and coach. He teaches mixed martial arts at Liberty University and is an assistant coach at The Edge Martial Arts. He is author of the Train Like a Pro book series, which also includes *Training for Mountain Biking: A Practical Guide for the Busy Athlete* (2021) and *Training for Obstacle Course Racing: A Pracical Guide for the Busy Athlete* (2021).

CPSIA information can be obtained
at www.ICGtesting.com
Printed in the USA
BVHW072354160521
607104BV00001B/2